"This book adeptly develops a numerical model to mathematize psychoanalytic impact on practice. This work distances number theory from quantification, and this will have an impact on analytic institutions and medical practices. It reflects on the urge to empirically quantify the results of psychoanalysis and offers an alternative model."

Arka Chattopadhyay, *Associate Professor of Literature, Philosophy and Psychoanalysis, IIT Gandhinagar, India*

"*The Mind of Complex Numbers and the Subject in Analysis* brings together, in a fluent manner, insights from mathematics, psychoanalysis and Buddhism, while anchored in up-to-date developments in physics and biology."

Anca Carrington, author, *The Unconscious as Space: From Freud to Lacan, and Beyond*

The Mind of Complex Numbers and the Subject in Analyses

In *The Mind of Complex Numbers and the Subject in Analyses*, Raul Moncayo uses the complex plane to evaluate analytic outcomes. Moncayo's approach provides a study of the process and outcomes of singular analyses that does not rely on the methods and questionnaires of psychotherapy or medical research.

Referencing topology and abstract mathematics, Moncayo explores the limits of the Cartesian plane for predicting the capacity for sublimation and positive outcomes. By integrating the complex plane, Moncayo arrives at an exact number to 'arithmetize' symptoms and human capacities.

This book represents a new approach to Lacanian analysis and outcomes that will be of great interest to Lacanian analysts in practice and training.

Raul Moncayo was born in Chile and first trained as a psychoanalyst in Buenos Aires. He obtained his PhD in social-clinical psychology at the Wright Institute in Berkeley and trained as an analyst at the Lacanian School of Psychoanalysis, which he also helped found. He is the founder of the Chinese American Center for Freudian and Lacanian Analysis and Research.

Routledge Focus on Mental Health

Routledge Focus on Mental Health presents short books on current topics, linking in with cutting-edge research and practice.

The Concept of the Individual in Psychoanalysis
The Ego, the Self, the Subject, and the Person
Raul Moncayo

A Critical Reconstruction of Evidence-based Practice in Psychology
Evidence and Ethics
Henrik Berg

Physician Wellness and Resilience
Narrative Prompts to Address Burnout
Pauline Davies and Cynthia M. Stonnington

Psychoanalysis and the Feminine
An "Other" Sex
Jacqueline Schaeffer, Translated by Andrew Weller

Efficient Therapy for Specific Client Problems
Making the Most of Every Client Session
Windy Dryden

The Mind of Complex Numbers and the Subject in Analyses
Raul Moncayo

For more information about this series, please visit: www.routledge.com/Routledge-Focus-on-Mental-Health/book-series/RFMH

The Mind of Complex Numbers and the Subject in Analyses

Raul Moncayo

Routledge
Taylor & Francis Group
LONDON AND NEW YORK

First published 2026
by Routledge
4 Park Square, Milton Park, Abingdon, Oxon OX14 4RN

and by Routledge
605 Third Avenue, New York, NY 10158

Routledge is an imprint of the Taylor & Francis Group, an informa business

British Library Cataloguing-in-Publication Data
A catalogue record for this book is available from the British Library

ISBN: 978-1-032-99986-9 (hbk)
ISBN: 978-1-032-99984-5 (pbk)
ISBN: 978-1-003-60703-8 (ebk)

DOI: 10.4324/9781003607038

Typeset in Times New Roman
by Apex CoVantage, LLC

Contents

Figures

Tables

Introduction

It is clear that the scientific aspect of language, is a maneuver of medicine, to psychitrify society like Laing Cooper, and Szasz, argued 40 years ago. In society, psychiatry has a veritable market of suffering. Many psychiatrists today charge $600 for a medication evaluation session and don't follow up with psychotherapy. Pharmaceutical companies gain enormous amounts of money from medications that otherwise help and are a help to psychotherapy.

Natural science considers psychiatry as a weak medical science that treats linguistic epiphenomena of brain processes. What brain processes? The pressure of drives, nervous impulses, emotions, thinking, and the inhibition of the same. Facilitation and inhibition are both physiological and mental. I argue that the wiring (writing) of the brain is an effect of the Mind, and that the Mind goes beyond the brain's determination because the Mind represents the brain's plasticity and capacity to change and evolve and go beyond the current brain.

It is well known that the training of every mental health clinician and medical doctor specialized in psychiatry involved a residency with applied theory and required interaction with psychiatrists, medical patients, and using diagnosis and medications.

I (Moncayo, 2018) have argued that Lacanian psychoanalysis has something to contribute to psychiatric diagnosis and treatment. It all begins with the theory of the signifier and using language, or the talking cure, and how mental signifiers differ from medical signs. Medical doctors read signs of the body/brain, while analysts read signifiers of the Mind. Psychoanalysis, in this book, includes an evaluation (diagnoses) and treatment of mental disorders and an outcome evaluation model based on abstract mathematics that is described in detail in the following pages.

The contribution of Lacanian theory to psychiatric and psychoanalytic diagnosis is its potential to simplify diagnosis without simplification. Instead of a flurry of postmodern multiplication of diagnosis and personality disorders, we only have three categories with three defense formations. Other diagnoses and personality disorders proliferate for the absence of theory and the fact that *Diagnostic and Statistical Manual of Mental Disorders, Fifth Edition* (*DSM-V*) abstains from it. The different personality disorders are not

DOI: 10.4324/9781003607038-1

structural differentiations but descriptive laundry lists of symptoms that can be understood in different ways.

For example, whether the person is schizoid or schizotypal is not that different, what matters is whether they are psychotic or neurotic, and if they are psychotic, do they have symptoms? Typically, the schizotypal has more symptoms than the schizoid, who can be confused with an introverted obsessional without social skills. The narcissistic personality is an exaggeration of hysteria, while the dependent personality is a feature of hysteria, and the avoidant personality is a subtopic of the obsessional structure. The histrionic is extroverted and likes to be the center of attention in a group. The obsessional structure is introverted, avoids the lack in relationships, and prefers to isolate with the ideal fantasy of their dreams.

Diagnoses also appear as symptoms that can or cannot be structures or surface formations. For example, a neurotic structure can have psychotic or perverse symptoms.

Finally, for Lacan phobia is a third form of neurosis, where the projected object unto the external world is not a forbidden object. The phobic object instead represents the father and symbolic castration. The father of little Hans could not lay down the law and separate him from his mother. Symbolic castration differs from the projected aggression of the bad breast, according to Klein, the loss linked to the phallus, differs from the loss linked to weaning from the breast.

I noted in my book on the practice of Lacanian analysis that Lacan utilized some notions in Freud (1933) about paranoia and the ego being formed out of early fixation and projection as a defense mechanism. I noted that Lacan was also a reader of Melanie Klein and the history of psychoanalysis. Lacanians who know Klein simply insert her model and use it within a larger Lacanian frame for the *objet a*. In this respect, Lacanian theory has respectfully subsumed but not denied Kleinian theory.

Metanoia refers to an early Greek concept developed by Jung (1961) but not found in Freud. Paradoxically, psychosis is a more severe condition than neurosis, but that, however, may overcome some of the problems of neurosis as Laing, Guattari, and finally Lacan argued. Lacan invented the concept of the sinthome to address what about psychosis is outside the oedipal structure, as Deleuze and Guattari argued. Using the four topological knots to describe the structures is an enduring contribution of Lacanian theory.

In the knot of three, the subject is socially bound by the signifier and the Name of the Father (NoF) coming from the Symbolic. "That by the fact of the said, they are arranged in a knot of three" (Lacan [1975–1976a], Session of 12.16.75, III 13). The statement both reveals and constitutes the knot of three under a conventional NoF that holds it together beyond Symbolic myths and laws. Instead, for the knot of four, it is the Real of jouissance that glues the knot together, not the Symbolic or the signifier. But the knot of three must be untied first.

Spaltung, or division into two (or more), simply refers to the division of the mind or personality accompanying or producing mental symptoms. How is it that the mind and the personality are divided into two rather than three? In fact, the mind is divided into two, but the two can become three because three come out of zero. Suppression represents the empty awareness that directs and suppresses experience. Today, *splitting* has acquired the meaning associated with normal neurosis in addition to a more severe division between the two that is unconscious. This, in turn, can refer to psychotic states (symptoms) or to structural psychosis without symptoms.

Freud's early studies of hysteria had many examples of seances and spiritism. This was Freud's Vienna. No wonder that the interest in the occult was prevalent at the time in the pre-Nazi Vienna. The Occult for Freud was the darkness of the house and the rooms of the unconscious. Jung, Freud's non-Jewish heir, took a different approach and thought of the unconscious here as the Shadow and gave it legitimacy as a form of knowing and intuition. This is the good darkness in contrast to the darkness of the id. Eastern darkness of Absolute non-knowing in which the agalma of awareness shines. Western darkness is the darkness and blindness of animal instinct. Lou Andreas Salome, Freud's student, represented the freedom of the phallus only in a phallic woman.

In the normal division of the subject, the division is accompanied by the symbol for money with two vertical lines of repression across the $ (one bar replicates into one or two). The bar indicates what the subject has lost, what is causing their desire, and, simultaneously, what is causing their lack.

This generates a schism that is not psychotic. The iconic form of projection that Freud considers is a neurotic form of projection, which he considers one of the defense mechanisms possible in psychosis. Somebody is projecting something onto you that doesn't belong to you.

Today, object relations analysts call projective identification, 'as-if' states, as if there are mental states of the analysand projected onto the analyst, who then experiences the projection within their own experience (the Bionian rather than Kleinian projection). Foreclosure, as we have said already, is a complete evacuation of the name of the father function within the symbolic order of language that otherwise exists despite the psychosis. The analyst works with their human subjectivity.

1 The Subject of the Real 'All-Alone'

Lacan's 'all-alone' is not the same as being lonely and isolated. In Genesis, G-d said that humans are not meant to be alone (referring to the problem between Adam and Eve, man and woman, yin and yang). But the religions expect priests and nuns to have an exclusive marriage with Buddha and Christ. Humans are not expected to live without G-d, whatever G-d represents: knowledge, love, meaning, order, and a partner. Everything in life is geared toward this aim. However, except in Japan, with its understanding of the implication or implicate order, Buddhist monks are allowed to marry other humans. In China, monks do not perform marriages or get married.

In Lacanian theory, there are three forms of the subject: the imaginary ego, the symbolic subject/signifier, and the Subject of the Real of jouissance. The symbolic Lacanian subject is different, and it is built based on the paternal Symbolic being a gateway to the Real, the directions in space lead you to deeper space without directions. Once you get there (material and mental space, visible or invisible), the lack in the Other is like a wormhole leading to Lacan's second Real. The signifier is both a subject and what of the subject is (signified) in the Real of jouissance left outside symbolization. The subject goes from hell to heaven. This outside runs not through Freud's ego but through the Kohut's and Winnicott's sense of a true self not as a concept but as an experience. This experience of jouissance and Real emptiness is the organization of emotional experience by pleasant and painful forms of jouissance:

> Frege founded the number one in the concept of inexistence. So, every material form that can be counted relies on the concept of inexistence or emptiness.
>
> The concept of inexistence differs from the concept of nothingness or emptiness. So in essence any form differs from itself by being nothing or empty rather than a specific form.
>
> (Lacan, 2016, p. 56)

The concept of emptiness used by Lacan is different than the Buddhist concept of emptiness. Lacan also speaks about true and false holes in the psyche.

DOI: 10.4324/9781003607038-2

This is similar to the concept of black holes in physics. Lacan, like Freud, used the physics of his time to build his theories of the psyche.

The asocial and 'trans social', as well as the social and transindividual individual, or the One, organize social experience for the Many in the interests of the Many. When the Many do not support the One, then the One cannot elevate the Many or the group. Conversely, when the leader or One is corrupted, Many are also corrupted.

2 Narcissism

> The substance of the subject Is the object substantiality is not of the subject itself but that of its objectified counterpoint, of an experimental and excremental reminder-trash which precisely sustains the subject qua empty and void and non-substantial subject. Do we have the empty unsubstantial subject precisely as such; however, it has to be sustained by a minimum of a pathological contingent stain, objet petit a. This object is the paradoxical stand-in for the Void of subjectivity; it 'is' the subject in itself in its otherness.
>
> (Zizek, 2000, p. 47)

Due to the absence of self, the *objet a* stands in for its absence. This is a brilliant idea of Zizek that I endorse. The subject is an object, and the object is a subject, but what about 'What' is neither? The subject of the real 'all-alone'.

Narcissism, Individualism, and Socialism

This image of a bubble represents the subject living in a One bubble with his/her biological environment. This is the subject of the Real. The notion that narcissism is a form of asocial egoism, is an ideological, not a scientific, concept that Bion used, and Lasch (1979) popularized it without including philosophy and critical theory. Early forms of narcissism are necessary for survival and healthy forms of self-love. Because an individual was loved by their mother in detailed ways, this also reflects an inspiring childlike love for others and beyond.

Alternatively, socialism can oppress natural talents in the service of hegemony or a homogeneous society, which will not make subjects happy. When the level of discontent among individuals reaches a massive critical point, then necessary social changes take place. The critical point may be on the critical line in the complex plane leading to nontrivial evacuations and returns to zero and the clean slate.

The brain functions in response to experience and yet experience is beyond brain function or cognitive thought and feeling. Especially with respect to the

DOI: 10.4324/9781003607038-3

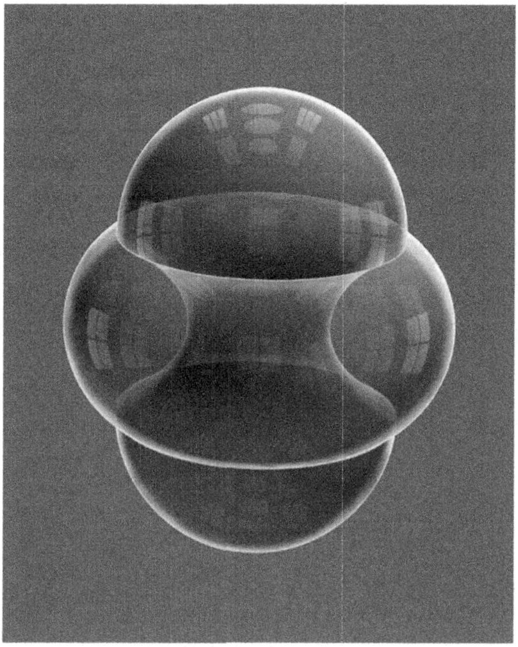

Figure 2.1 This image of a bubble represents the subject living in a One bubble with their biological environment

opening up of critical developmental periods in the brain (Robson, 2002), are these opening up periods, the time to structure the brain, or how the brain goes beyond the brain? The first is intuitive; the second, counterintuitive.

Language brings forth reality and the Real that is beyond language and the brain. Are Plato's solids not based on the existence of the brain? Of course not, because they are Mind or the forms of nature. Mind and the forms of nature are more than the brain, and as emptiness, Mind is more than form, including the forms of the brain.

At this level of ability, or function, IQ, translates to some molecule or level of electrical activity or magnetism. Repeated activity and electricity wire the brain. The windows or gateways of plasticity occur in different areas of the brain. In this sense, the structure of the brain is hierarchical (up or down like a tree) in the way that Piaget's developmental stages start with the frontal cortex and end with the serpent animal of the stem brain, from the concrete to the abstract, but then we have the nontemporal or eternal aspect of the structure, because the structure has existed before in time, although some formal elements may have changed and will continue to exist in the future.

Finally, we have the abstract concrete (the universe) and the concrete abstract (a pebble, a pearl, an electron, a monad, a pearl laughing at the bigness and power of the sun). From the concrete to the abstract are formal differentiations within logic, while the last two are non-dual differentiations within logic (not one/not two).

Otherwise, brain plasticity is only a mechanical engineering problem, rather than the more philosophical existential question of the human brain/Mind relationship. The brain, like the body, has repair processes. I ask, in turn, does the Symbol, or S, have repair processes? When the analyst listens to the contours of the voice of the signifier, the circling and cycling, between inside and outside, analyst and analysand, conscious and unconscious, is led by Tyche (the unconditioned opportunity) rather than automaton or repetition.

3 Is Psychiatry the Healing of the Mind or the Brain?

What is the electrical or magnetic component of brain plasticity? Well, our bodies themselves are electromagnetic. It is internal electrical activity that keeps our bodies magnetically alive. Our bodies naturally conduct electricity. In fact, every organ and cell in the human body has its own field.

The magnetic field produces electrical currents that are weaker than you may first think. At the same time, the electromagnetic field of the brain is stronger than the heart. Devices are able to measure the magnetic field created by the human brain. Despite how powerful it is, the magnetic field cannot harm the human body. The biomagnetic fields of the body, although extremely tiny, have been measured with techniques.

The body's electrical activity happens primarily in the cell membrane. It is tremendously important that the cell membrane maintains an appropriate 'charge' or voltage. A healthy cell has a transmembrane potential of approximately 80 or 100 millivolts. A cancer cell, for comparison, has a transmembrane potential often as low as 20 or 25 millivolts.

When the channels are closed, a cell membrane is at its 'resting potential' (calm mind), and when it is open, it is at its 'action potential'. Electrical fields are based on the buildup of electric charges in the environment. These electric fields are commonly associated with thunderstorms (brainstorm). The primary type of action potential is often referred to as the 'sodium-potassium pump', during which sodium flows into the cell via an entry channel and potassium flows out of a cell via an exit channel.

The brain has electro-neurostimulation, but what does the Mind have? The brain has 'excitement' cells or excitation whether joyful or excitable endocrine sexual cells. The answer is that, beyond the signifier, the Mind has magnetism, or the capacity to concentrate and create a field of serenity and tranquility, as in sleep (sleep is a conduit to hypnosis). The capacity to concentrate and the nerve impulses in the muscles, for example, the crossing of the legs in yoga, generate fast current pulses that induce a magnetic vacuum wave in the void of Mind.

It used to be believed that hypnosis and mental and emotional suggestion were due to unconscious magnetism, meaning that magnetism was like the

DOI: 10.4324/9781003607038-4

ether for the transmission of light and unconscious communication, which, finally, turned out to be wrong. If the source of magnetism was the ether and magnetism was related to the unconscious and sleep, then if there is no ether, what happens to the unconscious if there no ether?

The source of electricity and magnetism is light, so the medium of the unconscious is light/jouissance in the signifier and light as a signifier discerned in language. Jung said that there is light in the Unconscious. Through experiments, we clearly know that there is a division within the psyche between conscious and unconscious. In hypnosis, you give the subject an imperceptible suggestion that they do something, and they wake up and are compelled to do that, but they do not know why they are compelled to do that. Usually, if the subject is asked an extreme demand like committing suicide, they then awake from the trance and the natural trance of sleep.

If a person loses control of motor skills, as happens in fainting spells, seizures (accidental hysterical seizures), or dream paralysis, then this can be repaired not by identifying with a human but by identifying with ocean animal forms from which we came and identifying with water. This is very interesting and counterintuitive (unconscious intuition not conscious intuitive common sense). By imitating the movements of a dolphin in water, humans can reprogram the human brain by reopening the critical periods when new skills can be acquired.

Meditation does precisely this: opening the critical periods, which lead to emptiness and then to new understanding. We should teach this in school as a science not religion. Psychoanalysis may have a similar significant effect. Sessions open the Big Mind, which, in turn, opens the critical periods of the brain for healing and development.

4 Is the Brain Organized by Language or Mathematics?

Number is different from *quantity* and *large samples* in mathematics (Bateson, 1979, p. 53). Numbers are integers that can be counted with one's fingers. Uncountable numbers in the Cartesian plane, in extension, are only countable with a computer. Otherwise, uncountable numbers mean that the phenomenon of jouissance cannot be counted by numbers, one of the definitions of the Real opposed to the Real that can be accessed through mathematics.

This difference is basic for any sort of theorizing in behavioral science, for any sort of imagining of what goes on between organisms or inside organisms as part of their processes of thought in the brain. Numbers are the product of counting, and quantities are the product of measurement.

In 1980, I met Gregory Bateson at the Esalen Institute in the Carmel Valley of California. He was a scholar in residence and gave talks at night at in his bungalow. There were many people that night sitting on the floor. His theme was 'mental connections in the biosphere', how nature is 'mind', or mental-environmental, rather than brain. Now the study of the brain has revealed that the structure of the brain develops until age 5. This is similar to what earlier neurosurgeon Sigmund Freud said about mental development continuing to develop until the countable age of 5.

Bateson was giggling and laughing that night, and suddenly, the lights responded, flickering on and off, and objects started falling on the floor. The environment responded with electrical connection like the one running through the neurons of the brain. That was a better example than his logical mind could give.

These areas of the brain appear to be like the frontal cortex, the parietal lobe, and the occipital lobe. However, now we know that the frontal lobe is linked to the control of id-like emotional instinctual impulses. So, the ego would be in front, the superego would be in the place where the ego is in this drawing. What about the Occipital or 'reptilian' brain?

That numbers can be counted, conceivably means that they are more accurate because there is a discontinuity between each integer and the next. Between 2 and 3 there is a jump. In the case of quantity, there is no such

DOI: 10.4324/9781003607038-5

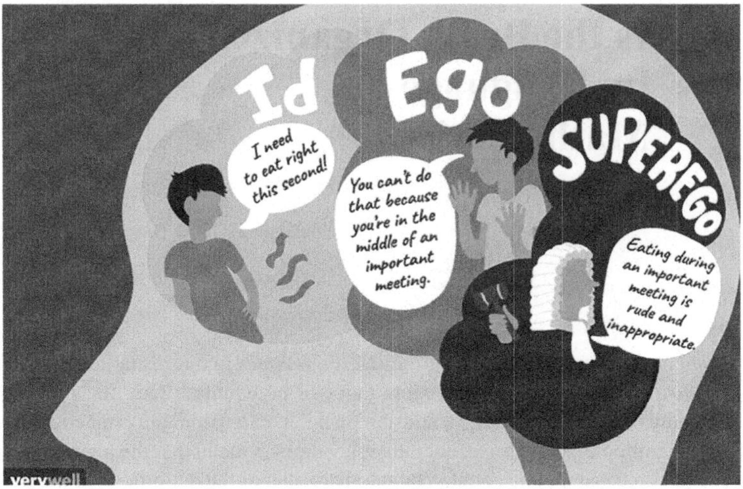
Id
Ego
SUPEREGO
I need to eat right this second!
You can't do that because you're in the middle of an important meeting.
Eating during an important meeting is rude and inappropriate.
verywell

Figure 4.1 The areas of the brain appear to be like the frontal cortex, the parietal lobe, and the occipital lobe

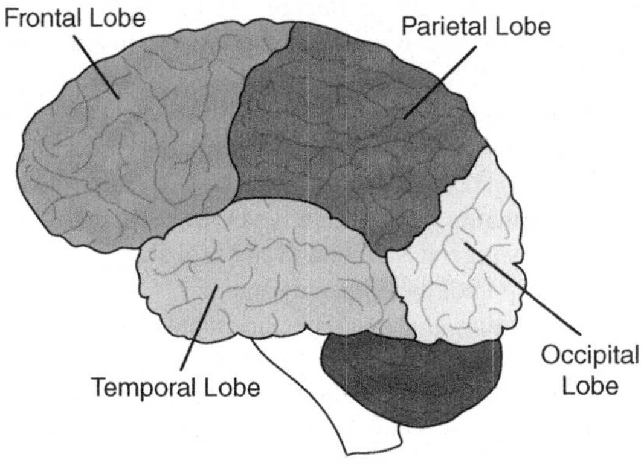

Figure 4.2 Brain lobe

jump, and because the jump is missing in the world of quantity, it is impossible for any quantity to be exact. You can have exactly 3 tomatoes. You can never have exactly 3 gallons of water. Always quantity is approximate. Even when number and quantity are clearly discriminated, there is another concept (pattern) that must be recognized and distinguished from both number and quantity period from this other concept of patterns whose members are commonly called numbers. Numbers are not numbers; sometimes, numbers are recognized as patterns.

Topology is a branch of geometry also defined by the existence of non-metric relations like numbers are. Topology, for example, was introduced by Lacan with a highly particular form of knotting: the Borromean knot. In Lacanian theory, you have to know at least how to count the four circles in the Borromean knot.

In Harari's (1995) book, he only recognizes phallic jouissance, the jouissance of the (m)Other, and the jouissance of meaning. The question follows as to whether the jouissance of the Other is imaginary while the Other jouissance is Real.

Numbers can be counted with the fingers but not large metric numbers that have to be counted by computers or artificial intelligence (AI). For example, if you want to study the experimental hypothesis that major depression is caused by the loss of a parent in childhood, you interview subjects and confirm that they had a loss of a parent in childhood. The small sample makes the information anecdotal data. Because the sample is small, we do not have to use probabilistic methods instead of a known rational sample. If the sample is too large, then probabilities and statistical methods are used.

But the psyche cannot be measured with large numbers only with numbers that can be counted with the fingers. It is like analysis. We only have small samples that report either failure or success in reducing symptoms. We can count the number of patients treated by any analyst. In addition, success is measured by increased sublimation and productive functioning.

People are knotted in knots of three at several levels. We have to disentangle the knot and tie a new knot. Symptoms are produced by knots, in what Lacan calls the sinthome, which is a new knot and a new name of the father.

People always have to enter analysis with symptoms of anxiety, depression, jealousy, anger, or envy. Some symptoms change with treatment, but some don't, or the subject does not want them to change, and they are part of their ego-syntonic personality.

To change symptoms, we have to differentiate between narrative speech and speech regarding the fantasy, and then finally, the analysis ends when the subject no longer needs the analyst. The analyst has become dispensable to the analysand.

5 Using the Complex Plane to Evaluate Analytic Outcomes and the Formation of the Brain

Instead of using large numbers to prove the effectiveness of psychoanalysis, or using numbers that can be counted with the fingers, we can use the complex plane instead of the Cartesian plane to evaluate analytic outcomes and the formation of the brain. In the complex plane, you find two kinds of Infinity, whereas in the Cartesian plane, you only find one form of infinity in extension. Complex intelligence is everywhere.

Preface

This book documents my practice of analysis over 25 years after years of training as a psychoanalytic psychotherapist and practicing in public and private settings. In contrast to my first book (2008), which failed to differentiate between hysteria and the borderline disorder, or between psychotherapy and analysis, this book only focuses on analytic cases. In addition, while my last book (2021) presented more female cases of hysteria, this book presents three male cases of obsessional neurosis and two cases of hysteria, one female case and one male case of hysteria, in the Lacanian sense.

I arrive at a way of quantifying psychoanalysis in mathematical and arithmetical terms that can be measured. I consider numbers that are symbolic elements appearing in dreams, fantasies, and narratives, as well as objective numbers observed in events.

As distinct from a quantity (see the following discussion) to 'arithmetize' symptoms and capacities, I distinguish among numbers, quantity, and images both sacred and profane. I arrive at an exact number/integer for the following:

1. The analysand's symptoms
2. The analysand's positive capacities
3. A number that measures and predicts the capacity to recover and traverse the fantasy
4. A number that measures and predicts the capacity for high realization and functioning.

DOI: 10.4324/9781003607038-6

Because this is not primarily a theoretical book, it includes the psychoanalytic literature that I have often cited in other work, insofar as I use previously established analytic concepts. I also include literature on analytic processes and outcomes. However, a clinical or practice book on method is now reformulated in this book as a mathematical discourse describable on the complex plane that measures the outcomes of psychoanalysis as a therapeutic practice.

This book presents a new approach that will be helpful to clinicians, analysts, supervisors, and administrators. It could be a federal model for mental health with stable long-term funding. This approach represents an effective clinical model for quality assurance and evaluating yearly outcomes, for example. I spent many years evaluating psychotherapy outcomes in a psychiatric clinic, not only to measure decreases in symptoms as a result of treatment but also to distinguish results that come from treatment and those that come from normal development and psychical resilience.

Epistemologically, psychoanalytic The American Psychological Association (APA) bureaucracies have regressed to statistical empiricism and reduced psychoanalysis to the large samples and statistical simplification that Freud rejected. Candidates in APA are asked about their treatment objectives with analysands. See, for example, Shendler (2010). Psychanalysis was waiting for a method to be invented to measure analytic effectiveness with a mathematical method consistent with psychoanalysis.

If you wait very long for a subject to change in analysis, they may change not because of analysis but because of the passing of time. Conversely, a subject is less likely to change in a short time, so if they change, it must be because of analysis and/or another accidental factor related to reopening critical periods in the brain. This points to the importance of transference cures at the beginning of analysis that motivate the analysand to stay in analysis and lose the money required for long-term refinance of painful personal debt.

Introduction and Methodology

This is a study of the process and outcome of singular analyses that does not rely on the methods and questionnaires of psychotherapy, or medical research.

Instead, I use abstract mathematics to make calculations that will not be based on large cardinal numbers emerging from large samples. Basic research uses probability research, for example, how many men or women suffer from depression and what type of depression. Instead, we list the symptoms as done in medical research. I want to prove the hypothesis that symptoms are cleared with the appearance of signifiers in analysis and their corresponding forms of pain and pleasure: jouissance. These signifiers, which often are names, are part of the unconscious signifying chain of a subject.

Applying the research done for a past book (*The Jouissance of Uncountable Numbers*, 2015), I consider research on the Cartesian plane, even if used for quantum research, only appropriate for measuring symptoms, not for predicting the capacity for sublimation and positive outcomes. I argue that the latter requires the complex plane to be measured. Most people are familiar with the Cartesian plane in science, but unfamiliar with the complex plane. The two planes share the x-axis and only differ by the i-axis. The i-axis is made of imaginary numbers that do not exist.

The following formula is our mathematical representation of symbolic castration, the central mathematical equation that organizes the theory.

Phi − phi = 1. The negation of the imaginary phallus: Phi − phi; 1.618 − 0.618 = 1 (Moncayo and Romanowicz, 2015). I dare say that this is the equivalent of Einstein's most important equation, although he was not a mathematician. This is our most important equation to characterize our use of mathematics to represent psychoanalysis. This formula is equivalent to the inhibitory function of the frontal cortex.

For each case, I arrived at a number based on both symbolic and arithmetical factors. A symbol comes out in a narrative, fantasy, or dream, and/or the number appears in symptoms and events. The imaginary that is empty, or does not exist in reality, is a measure of humanity in the good sense. The good or wholeness, or existential wholeheartedness, is the presence of emptiness that in the mathematics of the complex plane is reached through nontrivial zeros on the imaginary axis, which I make equivalent to the Buddhist emptiness as a whole. Trivial zeros are absences and deficits as shown in symptoms and appear on the Cartesian x-axis. I argue that jouissance requires quantum fluctuations in the void and that there are three of them. The first shows the farthest fluctuation from the absolute zero point as a state of constant excitation. The second has a closer fluctuation from the void, fluctuating between excitation and release. The third is closest to the zero of emptiness. My conceptualization relies on both mathematics and Mahayana Buddhism.

Because there are hidden (read substitutions) connections between numeric patterns/structures, not only new words or new numbers are produced by the function but also the phenomenological descriptions and elements, or shapes, found in biological forms and their variations, in planetary orbits and processes, and so on.

Instead of words, now we have worlds (astronomical, subatomic, biological molecular, cellular, viral, genetic). There are indeed numbers and logical connections embedded in biological forms. Since, for Freud, the id has been a biological substratum; perhaps he was wrong when in 1933 he said that "[t]he logical laws of thought do not apply in the Id and this is true above all of the law of contradiction" (the New Introductory Lectures, *SE*, 22, p. 73).

Contrast this with what Leibniz (1898; an earlier polymath) said in the *Theodicy*. To advance further, I want to return to the scientific work of Leibniz, a thinker who was overshadowed by Newton, beating him to the publication of the calculus. Leibniz's work still undergirds the study of gravity because physics uses his notation for Newton's theory of gravity. Leibniz anticipated the dialectical logic of Hegel but without grounding it in the pre-Socratics like Hegel and Heidegger did. Although Newton won the competition over the calculus with Leibniz, dialectical logic was a scientific discovery for Leibniz, not a historically based speculation as in Hegel.

Many judge philosophical theories in terms of idealism and realism. However, for a while now, I have argued that these categories do not apply today. Ideas are based on reality, and the Real is not reality, although all ideas come from the Real. Reality is based on images and language, and the Real is beyond both. Wrap your head around that knot.

> Our reasonings are grounded upon two great principles, that of contradiction, in virtue of which we judge false that which involves a contradiction, and true that which is opposed or contradictory to the false: (*Theodicy*, 44, 169). And that of sufficient reason, in virtue of which we hold that there can be no fact real or existing, no statement true, unless there be a sufficient reason, why it should be so and not otherwise, although these reasons usually cannot be known by us.
>
> (*Theodicy*, 44, 196)

> There are also two kinds of truths (something Nagarjuna invented the IAD): those of reasoning and those of fact. Truths of reasoning are necessary, and their opposite is impossible: truths of fact are contingent, and their opposite is possible. When a truth is necessary, its reason can be found by analysis, resolving it into more simple ideas and truths, until we come to those which are primary (nice description of free association).
>
> (*Theodicy*, 170, 174, 189, 280–282, 367)

It is thus that in speculative mathematics, Theorems are reduced by analysis to Axioms that are simple concepts, of which no definition can be given (i.e., emptiness); there are also first principles, which cannot be proved, and indeed have no need of proof; and these are identical propositions, that arise together with their opposites. (*Theodicy*, 36, 37, 44, 45, 49, 52,121–122, 337, 340–344.)

The truth value of Freud's statement regarding the id belongs to the logical level of impulse as experienced by a subject in society. A subject may follow the directives of the laws of desire (I want what I do not have and do not want what I have) or the law of the biological organism (hunger, for example), but the equations for these latter two conflict with the equation of what constitutes logical action in society (to use a trivial yet relevant example: to pee [p] or not pee [−p] in public).

There are numbers and logic at work in irrationality and irrational numbers despite the fact that what those numbers may represent in action may contradict what society considers logical according to other perhaps equally mathematical criteria. The irrational is not irrational but rather refers to a different form of rationality that denies the first and vice versa.

It is not the case that there is a logical system facing or interacting with another non-logical emotional system (this is only true at a phenomenological, descriptive, or existential human level). Rather, it is a matter of different logical types or levels, different levels of negation, and contradiction and non-contradiction. It is not a question of negation and no negation or a denial of negation; it is a matter of different forms of negation: unary and binary. I believe that the concept of unary negation is one of my contributions to the field, although it is the reissuing of an ancient concept.

In unary negation, the negated remains unmarked, thus giving the impression that 'nothing' has been negated. An act or a representation has been negated, and the void or absence left in its wake can also be negated or replaced with a new representation. What was negated is unconscious, and the unconscious appears as a void or a false hole, which itself can be negated. In a unary negation, what is negated is repressed or void, while in a binary negation, the negated is intellectually and consciously accepted.

Things, for example, can be perceived as numbers or sound waves, as music or noise, as pleasing or harsh. A harsh sound may produce a so-called irrational response such as fight or flight, attack or defend, and this may contradict a harmonious or pleasant response to sound, but in either case, a sound wave will be involved that under certain numeric conditions may produce contradictory (chaotic) or non-contradictory results (agreement or harmony).

I have shown how a function, or the Sense function can function in language and numbers. In language a function can work as sense or meaning, the latter includes censorship as a code (i.e., erase particular words/values from speech or writing) and can also be used to construct sentences and propositions. Sense or function can also be mathematical or arithmetical and refers to functions within numbers (i.e., multiplication of a number by itself). How Godel works up a code within numbers for numbers, as a form of self-consciousness.

Thus, the question can be raised whether there can be hidden connections not only between particular variables but also between the various codes at work in nature. The objects or inputs/outputs for the function may vary, although the function always transforms one into the other for various purposes associated with the various functions.

If prime numbers are the building stones of real numbers, then 2, the binary that postmodern thinkers hate, is the building block of reality. The first number is 1, but it is empty in its own being and therefore equals 0, as the first script and cipher. This is a Fregean counterintuitive foundation or axiom in mathematics like imaginary numbers are. The foundations of the Cartesian and complex planes are 2 and i, respectively.

The mathematically modeled Symbolic order consists of the triad of Sense or mental function, the arguments or the input/output of words/numbers and senses, and the sense objects that are apprehended by the structure as output. This is the 'what' of the structure and how the structure appears in the imaginary totality of visual perception.

Natural numbers appear to be ordered by logical or rational succession but, in fact, may be ordered by a ratio of irrational numbers, such as the golden number or pi, that continue to infinity. Mathematical structure does not exist in how numbers appear. You have to actually measure the shapes of nature and carry out arithmetical operations for the underlying so-called irrational ratio to appear.

In psychoanalysis, we do not perform arithmetical operations to reveal the irrational within the structure but, rather, use the rules of substitution and metaphor to arrive at the 'what' of the underlying structure that appears not to exist within the phenomenal or manifest figures of speech and discourse. In addition, the structure can also be said to not exist in that the structure is not the same as its instantiation in the phenomenal world and is not the same as the impossible and unnamable, which are actually what we are seeking in the search for truth and knowledge.

Of course, it all depends on how we measure effectiveness. This book offers an alternative scientific method to measure effectiveness in psychoanalysis. Finally, psychoanalysis has been repeatedly researched, yet its critics still claim that it is ineffective. Internally, its frequency has also been researched, and the study found no difference between two or three sessions per week and four or five sessions a week (Toronto, accessed 2023). The Lacanian school in America made psychoanalysis more effective and financially affordable by accepting two to three sessions a week, rather than the five to six a week as practiced by the International Psychoanalytic Association (IPA).

In analytic institutes, there are many who consider psychoanalytic psychotherapy more effective than psychoanalysis. Meta-studies also confirm the results obtained in other studies. However, post-analytical results continue to produce results way after the analysis has ended, thanks to Lacan's sinthome (I would add).

The Egyptian and Chinese Unconscious

For many years, scholars, and interested people, have been involved in an ideological controversy. Is Eastern culture collectively oriented, while the West is individualistic? Does Western psychology only apply to Europeans, or does the East have a unique manifestation of the Unconscious, or unique complexes, as some have argued? This book argues that both are true.

Freud saw psychoanalysis and dream analysis as an archeology of the mind. Therefore, in all languages, we find vestiges of other languages; in cultures, we find vestiges of other cultures; and in people and animals, we find vestiges of other beings. It is no surprise to discover that we find vestiges of Egyptian symbols in Chinese analysands, the two oldest cultures in the world, and of the history of the symbolic order, as I have called it. In all cultures, there are rudiments of mathematics and prime numbers, as seen in the examples of the Ishango bone in Africa.

The structure of language, and the structure of history, is much larger than the structure of cultures and nations. Larger structures determine how different myths manifest in different cultures, more than how humans build structure in history. This is true if only because atomic and subatomic matter and particles, all the way up in steps to molecules and then to organisms, demonstrate the same structure.

This book demonstrates the effectiveness of Lacanian psychoanalysis. Issues of confidentiality are uppermost in analysis, although Freud thought that scientific discoveries are more important than issues of confidentiality. However, the practice of analysis across cultures opens fresh new challenges. The question of names is fundamental for Lacanian analysis, and they have to be analyzed despite issues of confidentiality.

Treatment of the Obsessional and Hysterical Structures

Of the six cases first discussed, three are obsessional and three hysterical. We remind the reader that for Lacan these two diagnostic structures are defined by existential questions: 'Am I a man or a woman?' 'Are you a man or a woman?' The same logic applies to the question: 'Am I dead or alive?' Both structures always have symptoms and traits of the Other structure. This definition of *hysteria* differs from the *DSM*'s and Freud's. The latter define diagnoses by symptoms, not questions. This is the outcome of Lacan's interest in phenomenology and the existential tradition (Sartre [atheistic] and Heidegger [nontheistic]).

Obsessional structures cannot be treated directly (pure hate) and must be 'hysterized' in the transference. The three obsessionals were successfully hysterized in the transference, while the hysteric becomes more reflective, organized, and sober. The successful 'hysterization' of the transference leads to successful treatments. The failed cases do not have to be hidden to present a successful form of treatment for mental disorders. At any point in the method, the choices are clear that lead to failed treatments. You have to be able to explain why you fail and why you succeed. An explanation that is not an uninformed opinion is episteme, Sophia, and Nous.

The borderline condition also needs to be 'neuroticized' first before analytic treatment of a neurotic can begin. The borderline becomes a neurotic rather than a psychotic or pervert and is prevented and compelled from acting out. This would require a prior treatment of psychoanalytic psychotherapy where the focus is on the first phase of the Oedipus complex and the relation to the mother's jouissance and the refusal of the paternal function.

For this chapter, I use the complex plane to trace the path of the subject through analysis. The complex plane can answer the question, 'How did the therapeutic effect take effect on the subject?' The question of the symptom answers the question, 'What changed in analysis?' I measure symptoms in real numbers, and the capacity for sublimation is measured in imaginary numbers. Imaginary numbers allow us to see the deeper dimensions of reality such as the Buddha nature rather than simply nature.

In the past, psychoanalysis was rejected for being unscientific and for misusing the physics of the time. The rest of psychology relied on the experimental method, but more recently, psychology has relied on questionnaires and interviews. Each answer is scored from 1 to 5; the higher the number the closer it is to 1 as the truth, and most studies in medicine reach a margin of 0.025 of truth. The results are represented on the Cartesian plane. However, I argue that for psychoanalysis its efficacy is better represented by the complex plane with i numbers.

For each case, I arrive (based on counting) at a metaphor, a number, and a formula to describe the subject.

In the first case, for example, his anxiety, depression, and paranoia changed. What were the signifiers that emerged in his analysis that led to the resolution of his symptoms? I argue that in some cases, symptoms change and decrease as a consequence of the treatment, not only due to the passing of time. Ordinarily, symptoms are measured in the clinic with simple scales. The capacity for sublimation also plays a factor in the recovery from the symptoms. 'Arithmetized', the two give us a number for the subject. Imaginary numbers have to be reduced to and revealed through the Cartesian x- and y-axes.

Table 5.1 organizes the case materials into seven categories, and I give examples while protecting confidentiality. The clinical materials are organized by themes and signifiers, rather than biographical data (which also include numbers). Signifiers are singular markers of the subject's experience, rather than the researcher's constructs, presented to the subject in the form of questions. I offer a rationale for the subject, or the analyst, to disclose the structure (disclose) as an aspect of the sinthome:

1. Symptoms
2. Signifiers
3. Numbers
4. Desire
5. Desire of the Other
6. Sinthome
7. Nomination

Symptoms represent both signifiers and numbers, desire is interlocked with the desire of the Other, and the Sinthome is established as a process of nomination. In this sense, the table of categories constitutes a signifying chain, a causal chain, organized around a hole. The table of categories is a signifying chain of dependent origination.

For the case of S, the logical structure of the fantasy follows different content but the same process, so I will keep the format the same. The same is the case for Mario's case as well.

Table 5.1 The Chinese Unconscious

Symptoms were addressed through psychotherapy	*Diagnoses Hysterical neurosis with obsessional s.*	*Numbers*	*Signifiers are rank-ordered text*	*Desire is either 1, or signficant, or 0, or repressed*	*Desire of the Other is 1, or determining, or 0, or insignificant*	*Sinthome oIn i axis. Capacity for sublimation Level l of Emptiness Scale 0–10i His score: 2i*	*Nomination new name of the subject or the name is resignified in analysis*
1. Narcissism 2. Irritable 3. Depressed 4. Hypomanic 5. Insomniac 5 × 2i Measure of pathology and capacity for sublimation			1. Virginia 2. Gigolo 3. Hole 3. Imaginary phallus/wand 4. Mathemes for his symptoms 5. Circumcision 6. Ectonian phallus/ pregnancy 7. Government official				Grandpa Hao yu Grandpa Mu

Signifiers are different from symptoms, because they form part of the unconscious signifying chain associated with the name and nomination. Symptoms are described in a simple social narrative with gaps and omissions that point to the background signifying structure.

I arrive at a metaphor and a number for each subject.

The subject's metaphor is Grandpa Wu. Wu is not only no or lack but also the function of a unary negation. Wu in Chan means both no and yes.

The complex number of the subject is $2 \times 2i$.

The symptoms have lessened, although the subject began analysis with a medium capacity for sublimation. The score number is 2 in real numbers and 1 in imaginary numbers. His complex number during treatment is $2 + 2i$.

For purposes of clarity, I write and view his complex number in a binary matrix. Matrix mathematics is a branch of mathematics used by Dirac to reconcile relativity theory with quantum physics. The numbers here represent the analysand (a possible card in a deck of cards), not subatomic particles and the exchangeability of electricity and magnetism. Here I am speaking of the exchangeability of suffering and drives for sublime ideals and the assigning of a specific number to a subject. A number 2 is assigned to pathology on the reality axis and a number $-2i$ to 'desublimation' on the imaginary axis. Marcuse's desublimation is a measure in the negative quadrant of imaginary numbers.

6 Complex Numbers Shown in Binary Matrixes Treatment of the Obsessional and Hysterical Structures

Of the six cases discussed, three are obsessional and three hysterical. We remind the reader that for Lacan these two diagnostic structures are defined by the questions, 'Am I a man or a woman?' 'Are you a man or a woman?' The same logic applies to the question, 'Am I dead or alive?' Both structures always have symptoms and traits of the Other structure. This definition of hysteria differs from the *DSM*'s and Freud's. The latter define diagnoses by symptoms, not questions.

Obsessional structures cannot be treated directly (pure hate) and must be 'hysterized' in the transference. The three obsessionals were successfully hysterized in the transference, while the hysteric becomes more reflective, organized, and sober. The successful hysterizing of the transference leads to successful treatments. The failed cases do not have to be hidden to present a successful form of treatment for mental disorders. At any point in the method, the choices that lead to failed treatments are clear. You have to be able to explain why you fail and why you succeed. An explanation that is not an uninformed opinion is episteme, Sophia, and Nous.

Now the difficulty with hysterizing one of the obsessional structures in the sample of cases is that he had a particular conflict or fear of being feminized. So, being seductive with him, and being a male analyst, he could interpret the 'hysterization' as a homosexual seduction. What protected this particular analysand from that fear was a symbolic identification with psychoanalysis and Freud.

In this chapter, I use the complex plane to trace the path of the subject through analysis. The complex plane can answer the question, 'How did the therapeutic effect take effect upon the subject?' The question of the symptom answers the question, 'What changed in analysis?' I measure symptoms in real numbers and the capacity for sublimation in imaginary numbers.

For each case, I arrive at a metaphor, a number, and a formula to describe the subject.

DOI: 10.4324/9781003607038-7

In the first case, for example, his anxiety, depression, and paranoia changed. What were the signifiers that emerged in his analysis that led to the resolution of his symptoms? I argue that in some cases, symptoms change and decrease as a consequence of the treatment, not only due to the passing of time. Ordinarily, symptoms are measured in the clinic with simple scales. The capacity for sublimation also plays a factor in the recovery from the symptoms. 'Arithmetized', the two give us a number for the subject.

A table organizes the case material into seven categories. I give examples while protecting confidentiality. The clinical material is organized by themes and signifiers, rather than biographical data. Signifiers are singular markers of the experience of the subject, rather than constructs of the researcher, presented to the subject in the form of questions. I offer a rationale for the subject, or the analyst, to disclose the structure (disclose – not advertise) as an aspect of the sinthome.

1. Symptoms
2. Signifiers
3. Numbers
4. Desire
5. Desire of the Other
6. Sinthome
7. Nomination

Symptoms represent both signifiers and numbers, desire is interlocked with the desire of the Other, and the sinthome is established as a process of nomination. In this sense, the table of categories constitutes a signifying chain, a causal chain, organized around a hole. The table of categories is a signifying chain of dependent origination.

For the case of S, the logical structure of the fantasy uses different content but the same process, so I keep the format the same. The same is used for Martin's case as well.

Signifiers are different from symptoms because they form part of the unconscious signifying chain associated with the name and nomination.

I try to arrive at a metaphor and a number for each subject.

The subject's metaphor is Grandpa Wu. Wu is not only no or lack but also the function of a unary negation.

The number of the subject in the complex plane is $2 \times 2i$.

The symptoms have gone down, although the subject began analysis with a low capacity for sublimation. The score number is 2 in real numbers and 1i in imaginary numbers. His complex number during treatment is $2 + 2i$.

Table 6.1 Chinese Case

Symptoms were addressed through psychotherapy	*Diagnoses Hysterical neurosis with obsessional sx.*	*Numbers*	*Signifiers are rank-ordered in the text*	*Desire is either 1, or significant, or 0, or repressed*	*Desire of the Other is 1, or determining, or 0, or insignificant*	*Sinthome on i-axis Capacity for sublimation Level of emptiness $0–10i$ His score: $2i$*	*Nomination new name of the subject or the name is resignified in analysis*
			1. Virginia				Grandpa Haoyu
1. Narcissism			2. Gigolo				Grandpa Mu
2. Irritable			3. Hole				
3. Depressed			3. Imaginary phallus/wand				
4. Hypomanic			4. Mathemes for his symptoms				
5. Insomniac			5. Circumcision				
			6. Ectonian				
$5 \times 2i$ Measure of pathology and capacity for sublimation			7. Government official				

For purposes of clarity, I write and view his complex number in a binary matrix. Matrix mathematics is a branch of mathematics used by Dirac to reconcile relativity theory with quantum physics. The numbers here represent the analysand, not subatomic particles and the exchangeability of electricity and magnetism. Here I am speaking of the exchangeability of suffering, drives for sublime ideals, and assigning a specific number to a subject. A number 2 is assigned to pathology on the reality Cartesian axis and a number −2i to 'desublimation' in the imaginary axis.

Repressive desublimation, a term first coined by Frankfurt school philosopher and sociologist Herbert Marcuse in his 1964 work *One-Dimensional Man*, refers to the way in which, in advanced industrial society (capitalism), 'the progress of technological rationality is liquidating the oppositional and transcending elements in the higher culture.' The higher culture is getting desublimated. Finally, the discourse of the capitalist is the discourse in which the subject completes themselves through consumption, and the science and knowledge about the objects of consumption also lead to increased consumption. Lacan calls the *objet a* a 'lathouse' to refer to the use of computers and internet-based information and AI to impact consumption and economic exchange. The information about the *objet a* is Imaginary, but it facilitates economic exchange.

Continuing with his formula,

$$\begin{pmatrix} 2 & -2i \\ 2i & 2 \end{pmatrix}$$

$$(2+-2\mathrm{i})\times(2\mathrm{i}+2)\rightarrow(4+4\mathrm{i})\cdot$$

In this case, the subject's complex number is 4 + 4i emerging from the core of their being, or, in other words, the core of the axis. Complex numbers have a wave function from 2, −2 to 4, −4, and so on.

Maxwell used matrix mathematics to describe the exchangeability of electricity and magnetism. To obtain a single matrix equation instead of a pair, new functions were constructed using the components of the Riemann–Silberstein vector. For Riemann (1854), geometry is about calculating the length of every curve. It is unclear to me how the study of spheres and circles was a mystical concern of Pythagoras in antiquity that continued into the Middle Ages, but somehow modern geometry is different from that? It turns out that the new geometry is very much like the old geometry and calls out the outlines and limits of coastlines and the shapes of leaves 'as if' out of nowhere.

I am sure that this statement reflects my ignorance of how the two geometries understand triangles and angles differently. Nevertheless, I use matrix mathematics to describe the exchangeability of the signifier, for images, and for images for jouissance. $(S \rightarrow I \rightarrow R = X \rightarrow Y \rightarrow Z)$. RSI (Real, Symbolic, Imaginary) is the function of XYZ.

Jouissance has acceleration in the displacement from signifier to signifier, while jouissance can also be condensed in a metaphor. Conversely, magnetism can be condensed in a chain of metaphors or can represent the condensed Real beyond or outside representation. Is the radiation associated with magnetism damaging or medically therapeutic? Using radiation in war is damaging, while in a small dose, it is positive. Positive and negative charges repel each other, and this is how magnetism controls for gravity.

Is there anything spiritual about magnetism? Is magnetism the mind equivalent of the concentration of samadhi or even the Sabbath (*Samedi*)? It all depends on the color (quantity) of energy concentration (blue is cool and low entropy, heat is red, and the spectrum between these two colors is purple). Nirvana is blue and cool, and fire and light are pure energy, yellow and red, respectively. Purple is the color of nobility of spirit. Blue is calm, and red is passion and compassion. Magnetism is what stops you when you move or fall (think of a free climber depending on the magnetism between their fingers and the fractal shape of the mountainside). Stopping is the same as calmness of mind and non-movement. You stay calm because you do not move, and because your body-mind does not move, you can travel fast. The universe is accelerating, and at the same time, it does not move and stays in the same place.

Cxyz is the complex subjugation of SIR into the quantifying triplet, and $M = [M_x, M_{y,} M_z]$ is a vector whose component-permuting elements are abstract as 4×4 matrices have shown. We have RSI, ISR, SIR, SIR, and the sinthome.

From the component M-matrices, we get

$$\Omega \quad \begin{matrix} [0 & -I_2] \\ [I_2 & \mathbf{o}] \end{matrix}$$

$$\beta \quad \begin{matrix} [2i & 0] \\ [0 & 2i]] \end{matrix}$$

Alpha (the center of the *x*- and i-planes) and Omega represent the wave function and the infinite straight line emerging from the center of the plane which is the objective equivalent of the subjective center of a subject.

The subject of the complex plane is both a subject and an object in a dialectical moment as Freud, Jung, and their followers believed.

We see in following figure that the complex plane looks like the Cartesian plane, except that the numbers differ and signify the different circles, which represent symbolic positions.

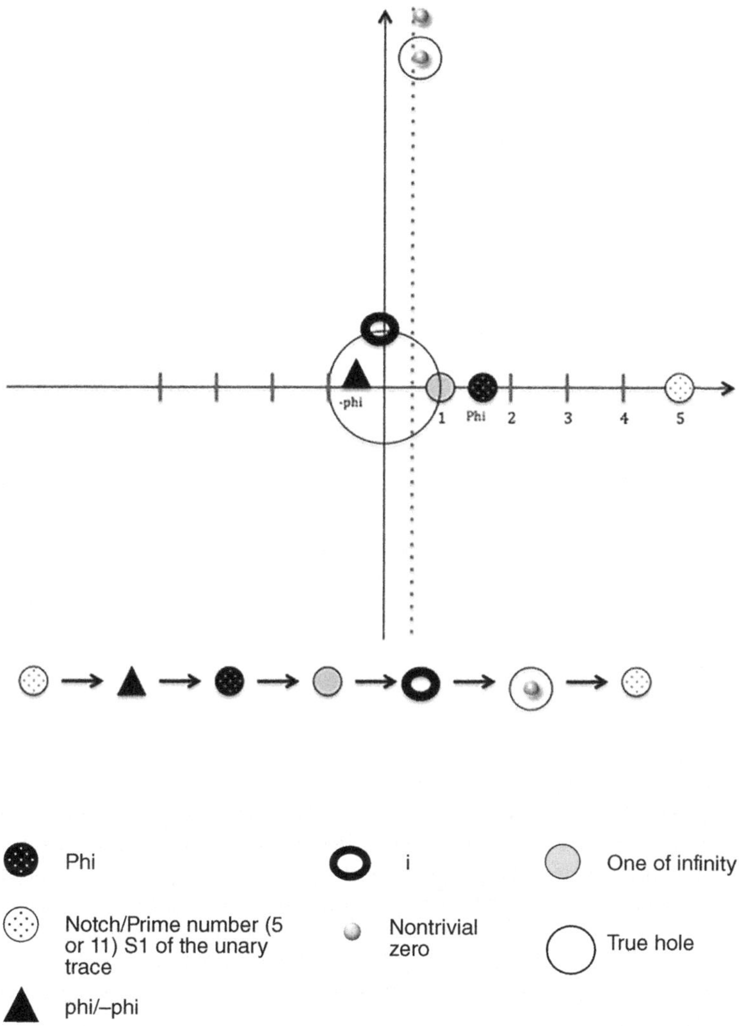

A tensor in physics, for example, has four component elements, revealing a formal structure and order at the microparticle level. Ordinarily, the macro level represents order, and the micro level represents disorder. Here, the micro is orderly while the macro is disorderly. What are the implications of this? Well, usually the small, or the leader, is controlled by the large, although the subjective experience of the leader and group members may be the reverse. In this case, however, the large, or the group, is also controlled by the leader or the small. For psychoanalysis, the small is the *objet a*, expressed as a tensor. Why is the *objet a* organizing rather than disorganizing? Rotation around a centripetal hole, for example, structures the elliptical orbits of the planets. A tensor is effective in counting the sexual tension inside a subject in relation to the object causing desire.

The micro is like the order of RSI installed at a microparticle level with 0 and 1 as imaginary numbers, in addition to the 0 and 1 of real numbers. The fourth element I name the third jouissance, a convenient positive feeling state or sense of well-being that is immeasurable and nonnumerical (1 = R).

There is a positive and a negative 1. The Real is the 1 that is 0 or a 0 that is a 1. The Imaginary is the 1 that is 1. Then there are also two zeros: the zero of absence and the zero of presence. Zero is the signifier of desire and lack (S); 0′ is suffering or pain, as a negative absence (Imaginary −phi or −0.68 . . .), and another 0 as a sense of well-being derives from emptiness.

From 0 as a signifier of desire or lack, and the imaginary phallus as a virtual source of suffering, for Lacan, the ψ phallus also appears as a golden number in the form of 0.68. In the matrix, the phi could also be represented as a temperature or heat tensor and how a vernacular use of language links heat to sexuality. A heat tensor for a subject would pair the heat of the drive (nature) with the heat of ideals (the burning bush) in the biblical burning bush.

$$(4 \times 4i)$$

$$(-4i \quad 4)$$

These four elements also correspond to the four levels of the signifiers: the trace/trait lower unit of the signifier, the letter, the word, and the sentence. The four positive and negative elements interact within the matrix, generating the formal structure of the thinking that determines the subject's experience, as well as the outside that organizes the order and cohesion of the structure. Here the theory is formally modeled after mathematics, but the arithmetization still has to be proven by being replicated and validated by real mathematicians. My use of abstract mathematics, although accurate, is intuitive or philosophical but is not a mystical use of numbers as in Jewish or Christian gematria and/or numerology.

The 1 in the matrices are imaginary numbers. What does it mean in this model that sublimation is described by imaginary numbers that do not exist? In addition, the 0s can be the 0 of the Cartesian plane or the 0 of the complex plane. This real 0 also differs from the nontrivial 0s that appear in the critical line (0.5) along the i-axis of imaginary numbers. Trivial 0s appear on the real x-axis.

Sublimation is a different negativity (−1) than the negativity of negative x numbers in the Cartesian plane. Sublimation is a positive negativity that differs from repression or is a different type of repression. Sublimation is based on a primary form of repression in the Real unconscious that is not oppressive. We do not know 'it' or repress/forget it because it is a Real outside representation.

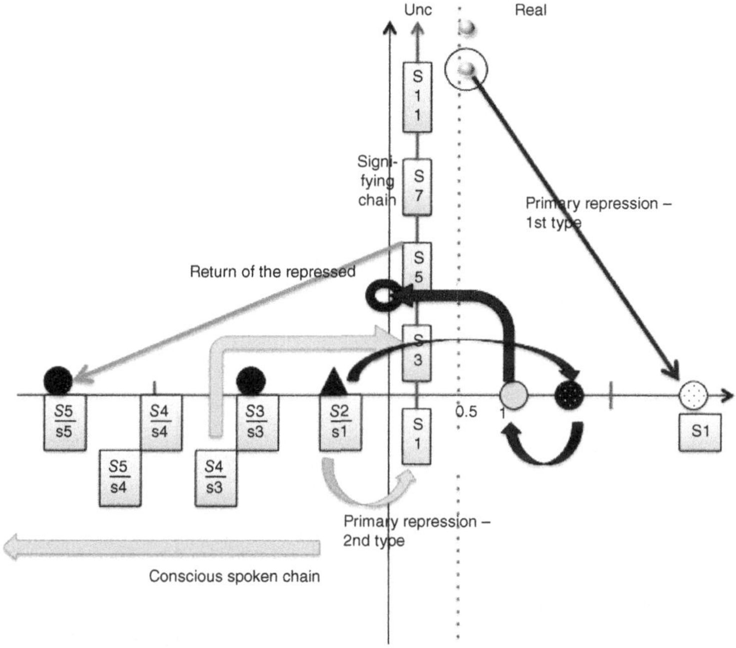

In the case of this Chinese subject, the i of imaginary numbers is low, or a small number, as shown in this graph. We see that in the negative x-axis the numbers come in pairs of signifier/signified. On the positive side of the x-axis, prime numbers appear. In our cases, only two cases generated the prime numbers 5 and 7. Prime numbers are what build structure, so these case examples happen to be of leaders in a field of knowledge.

Case of S

Symptoms	*Diagnoses*	*Ranked signifiers*	*Numbers Total 6*	*Desire 1 or 0*	*Desire of Other 1or 0.*	*Sinthome*	*Nomination*
1. Depression	Obsessional neurosis with hysterical symptoms	1. My son the doctor 2. My son the criminal		1. To be a man. Fuck 1 or 2	1. That he be a man	He is a sinner/saint who 'fucks' paternal grandmother (2 1i) (1i 2)	the One who bears
2. Anxiety		S. the snake, the player		Kill the father steal the breast			
3. Fear 4. Being minority 5. Paranoia							

The subject's metaphor: the One who bears.

His complex number after treatment is $1 \times 2i$.

Formula for the subject: The complex number read as a binary matrix and represented in a graph:

$$\begin{pmatrix} 1 & -2i \\ 2i & 1 \end{pmatrix}$$

$$(1+-2i)\times(2i+1)\rightarrow(2+4i)$$

Complex numbers convert the false hole into the true hole, the emptiness of absence into the emptiness of presence, and calculate the level of emptiness (depression) and the level of sublimation. Take, for example, a subject with symptoms yet a high spiritual or aesthetic capacity for sublimation in art or mathematics.

Case of Martin

Symptoms	*Diagnoses*	*Ranked signifiers*	*Numbers*	*Desire*	*Desire of Other*	*Sinthome*	*Nomination*
1. Anxiety	Hysterical neurosis with obsessional symptoms	My son the bohemian		1. To be a woman	He has to account for himself. That he be special	He is a sinner/ saint pervert who wants to kill his father	The Martyr
2. Malevolent depersonalization							
3. Addiction							
Complex score 3 × 2i		After treatment 1 × 2i Psychoanalysis is the ideal but is no longer idealized	1 Not a prime number, although it is the origin of numbers			2i	

Metaphor of the subject: the Martyr.
Number for the subject is $3 \times 2i$.
Formula for the subject:

$$\begin{pmatrix} 1^{\cdot} & -2i \\ -2i & 1 \end{pmatrix}$$

$$(1+-2\mathrm{i})\times(-2\mathrm{i}+1)\rightarrow(2+-4\mathrm{i})$$

Literary Benevolence

Symptoms	*Diagnoses*	*Ranked signifiers*	*Numbers*	*desire*	*Desire of Other*	*Sinthome*	*Nomination*
1. Anxiety	Obsessional structure with hysterical symptoms	1. peachy	3 and 7 = 10	1. little devil	That he be special boy 1	He is a sinner with women	1. son of the Buddha: Rahul 2. Moncayo. The name of a mountain in Spain.
2. Am I dead?		2. My son the handsome scholar 3. you shall amount to 'nothing' like my brother Augustus		2. To be a Buddha	He writes like the greats	Mystic third jouissance and jouissance of meaning	2.The empty mountain spirit of truth
Before treatment $2 \times 3i$	After treatment	$0 \times 7i$ 7i out of 10	7 Is a prime number				

Metaphor of the subject: the spirit of truth.
The number for the subject: 0 × 7i.
The formula for the subject:

$$\begin{pmatrix} 0 & -7i \\ -7i & 0 \end{pmatrix}$$

$$(0+-7)\times(-7+0)\rightarrow(0+-14\mathrm{i})$$

Case of M

Symptoms	*Diagnoses*	*Ranked signifiers*	*Numbers*	*Desire*	*Desire of Other*	*Sinthome*	*Nomination*
1. Anxiety	Hysterical neurosis with obsessional symptoms	My son the scholar. Traumatic mother's gaze takes son's picture	4	To be a boy 1	That he be special boy He completes both parents	He is a boy addicted to mother's breast	Yin The 'holy' dark light in your eyes
2. I am and my father is a woman						Feminine third jouissance	
2. I and father are crazy 3. Depersonalization 4. Addiction		$4 \times 3i =$ After treatment $2 + 4i$				3i	

The metaphor of the subject: The name as a light in a man: The 'holy' dark light in your eyes.

The number of the subject is 2 × 5i.

The formula for the subject

$$\begin{pmatrix} 2 & 4i \\ 4i & 2 \end{pmatrix}$$

$$(2+4\mathrm{i})\times(4\mathrm{i}+2)\rightarrow(4+8\mathrm{i})$$

The score of the treatment indicates the level of recovery and the potential for higher functioning. If the *x*-axis numbers remain high and the i numbers remain low, then the chances of change are also low.

The higher the i score, the higher the potential for the subject to be a successful professional, or analyst, a true teacher, or scholar. In this case, the subject is a senior analyst who has reached a 7 in a total score of 10. A total score of 10 would be unreachable perfection.

New name from the Real is resignified as 'in-you' because the name in Chinese also means 'in'. The other name means 'foreign' or 'out'.

The name is a symptom, the supplement of dependence on the man (male or female) to become a strong man like the problem with hysterical dependence on names to be strong. Now with the new name of 'in-you', you have a relationship to the name and the symbolic phallus in the form of the *objet a* as eyes as 'in-you' as a woman. The strength of the imaginary phallus that you lack, you search for in the dependence to the name or the man.

I am really impressed by your interpretation, Raul. No word can express my feelings at this moment. What I may respond is maybe 'It's just like this'. It seems that you find out that exact me in me. The other day you mentioned my family name as 'in-you'. I was impressed by your connection then because the sliding sound from 'in' to 'you' in English is very similar to the Chinese pronunciation of my name, and most importantly, the sound from 'in' to 'you' also corresponds to the exact meaning of 于 in Chinese, 'in something or related to something'. 'New Name from the Real' reminds me of Joyce and his mention of epiphany. Yes, this is a moment of epiphany for me. The new name from the Real is the NoF from the Real. Thank you for leading me there.

I was especially shocked by your interpretation of my symptom. You make what you said yesterday more clearly to me here. Thank you for that. Yesterday when you mentioned several names, I've already received the message. It produced a great therapeutic effect upon me. And I had a dream this early morning where my high school class teacher appeared. She shared the same name with my mom, a kind of flower. Yes, my name is always my symptom, symbolizing something problematic with the side of masculinity in me.

This is why Nan Huaijin (南怀瑾), a famous Chinese cultural scholar for I-Ching (易经) warned people not to study yin–yang philosophy. You helped me get an intimate touch with it. That is an amazing journey full of Lacan's detours and Godel's twists. But different from Nan Huaijin's worries, I believe that the destination is very clear: it will lead to more discoveries, beautiful and inspiring in every sense.

Phoneme is based on sound. 'In you' is like a sound that is like drawing a circle in the air that represents the wave of sound as a traceless trace that erases the trace of the symptom through a homophone. The wave of sound then is interpreted as 'just this' and 'just this' is represented as a form of the third jouissance. Russell said the first names like John or Mary means 'just this' as a singularity of jouissance rather than a particular person.

With the gaze and the eye, we also have a wave of light, so the light in you, that you get back from using me as *objet a* of the gaze. The eyes in you, the pearl in you that you saw in the form of the Other's gaze, comes back to you as inner light, or the inward light.

'Thank you very much, Raul, for the further explanation. phoneme is based on sound. In you is like a sound that is like drawing a circle in the air that represents the wave of sound as a traceless trace.'

Russell said the first names like John or Mary means 'just this' as a singularity of jouissance rather than a particular person. This part is quite mystic, Raul. But since you lead me to feel it more and more in analysis, I know what you are saying. It's a knowing upon non-knowing. It just happened. Words fail to explain it, but sound is so full at the moment. Sound is the intangible Real. It impowers the signifying chain to run only on the level of the signifiers by turning itself into phoneme and creating new signifiers, and in this way, the symptom as the signified inscribed in the body, is emptied of its meaning and therefore falls off from its original signifiers.

This analysand's symptoms were anxiety, jealousy, and envy for which I gave her −2i. Her abilities included high intelligence and spirituality, so I gave her 5i. Through analysis, her score went up from −2 to 3i. Her abilities helped her wake up in analysis to 6i.

Case of T

T is a very attractive 40-year-old highly educated professional woman self-described as a feminist.

The request for analysis was expressed in terms of her desire to understand what happened with the failure of her first marriage, seeking relief from the guilt she felt over this, and the problem represented by a very disturbed daughter of her current partner. She also reported a problem with a generalized sense of anxiety.

With her first husband, she married a man who was very successful, attractive, experienced, and very popular with women. Initially she said that the marriage failed because neither believed in fidelity, and the marriage ended when she left her husband for one of her lovers.

At the outset of analysis, she wanted to let me know that infidelity was not a problem for her, that she did not see it as a symptom, and that she justified it in terms of a feminist ideology that a woman's body is not a man's property. She was speaking to the Other, the father, who could judge her, lay down the law, or embody the guilt and the very much fought against a sense of debt toward her first husband. As is always the case in analysis, gradually in time, the story changes as hidden and censored details, fantasies, memories, and signifiers emerge. The no-law of the analyst emerges as the censored law operating within the subject.

T did not believe in fidelity, because the mother had suffered for her sexual fidelity to the father. Because of being faithful, her mother did not leave her father, although he was obnoxious, domineering, and right wing. But her father was lacking in intelligence and education. There was an imaginary father; there was also a symbolic lacking father, but it could not symbolize the lack in the father. Nor could she or her mother symbolize the lack in the mother because her mother was perceived as perfect and the father as unworthy. Had her father been educated then she could symbolized his lack, her mother's, and her own. She did not believe in tying herself down to any man. She was her own best man.

With her first husband, she did not feel pleasure, and she either felt nothing or sex was painful. He was a Don Juan type who wanted to show his sexual prowess, and although allegedly neither of them believed in marital fidelity, when she finally left him for her current partner, he became unglued to the point of suicidality and suicide threats. She also disliked the desire that he had for her recognition of his sexual and intellectual prowess.

Another thing that emerged in the course of analysis is that with some trepidation she disclosed that she never wanted to have children. Again, like with the question of fidelity, she did not want this seen as a symptom, although again when the law was not forthcoming from me, she wondered several times that maybe she should have children. As an explanation and justification for not having children, she quoted her mother who always told her that although she loved her and her brothers, she would have preferred to have not had children and dedicated herself to her career. Her father has asked her for grandchildren and often when she was an adolescent wanted her to be a decent girl and not a "prostitute" and not to wear miniskirts or stay out late; although when she did it anyway, he looked the other way. Her mother felt tied down to her father, who was considered a very good provider and sexual partner but a burden nonetheless. Her father was not educated, and her mother had a PhD. Her mother is described as more intelligent than her father. In addition, he had a bad temper and very right-wing political beliefs. He is said to have adored her mother and no complaints are given of her.

The reason T herself gives for not wanting children is due to all the service work required. However, another complaint was that she provided too much service to friends, coworkers, and others; was never able to say no; and was always being taken advantage of. In other words, service is a kind of jouissance to her. She met her current boyfriend when they were both married, and both left their spouses. He was married to a woman 15 years older than him and has a daughter who became severely anorexic, bulimic, a cutter, and suicidal with her parents' divorce. The daughter requires constant supervision, and the father is totally at her bequest and has reassured T that he will do all the work and that she will not have to do any. Now T is going to live with him, and so will the daughter, so T feels haunted by having to have a daughter she did not want and who requires an absolute form of service.

T's partner is loyal to her, but she has told him that she does not believe in fidelity, and he tolerates this but is not pleased. She describes their sexual relationship as very enjoyable, although when they are apart, she does not miss him and instead fantasizes about another man with the return of her partner being a spoiler of the party. However, she is very dependent on being loved by the boyfriend and does not want to leave him or be left by him. At times, she also expressed the desire that her partner would limit her excess. Recently, she met a younger man who did not succumb to her advances, and this was very destabilizing for her. Every now and then, she comes to her sessions with microskirts, and she lifts her legs while on the couch.

Recently, with much embarrassment and reluctance to explore and associate with the material, she disclosed that during sex, they role-play her fantasies where he is with another woman or she is with another man or where she is another anonymous woman who sometimes is a prostitute. The disclosure of these fantasies was prefaced by apologies and justifications that fantasies are a normal part of the sexual relationship. In other words, fantasies sustain desire. However, the way that fantasies are symptoms that defend against castration is not something that she yet can consider.

She further disclosed with vulnerability and without apology or justification prostitution fantasies, which are masturbatory in nature, where she is a prostitute to a line of men who want her service, and she very much wants to satisfy all their fantasies and desires.

In a dream, T is with many naked men; among them is her ex-husband. He has an erection, but the penis is facing down. She then begins to spin like Clark Kent does to turn into Super-Man and becomes a superwoman.

Associations: She is one of the men. She always likes being among groups of men and feeling like she is one of them. Cartoon of a little girl who transforms into a supergirl or heroine. The lowered erection makes it less threatening and intrusive. The inverted male sign is a symbol used by feminists. During puberty, she was embarrassed about having breasts, and she would wear special clothing to disguise them. Growing up, she wanted to be a boy and not a girl. She did not want to have breasts, did not play with dolls, and was a tomboy. She had a profound disgust and fear of menstruation.

Termination

Feelings and thoughts about it. No, will work on it with Hans in Mexico. Her analysis will not end because she will continue with her self-analysis. The other is not symbolized. The other is either replaced by a substitute or by herself. She talks about herself but not to me. Or she talks to me but not about herself but about me and my shortcomings. For example, when she referred to my speaking too much or more than her previous analyst or how she liked an analyst in Mexico. This is the place of the analyst as the man who "*no sirve*" (it is useless), good for nothing, Lacanian analysis does not work or does not function, is impotent. Then there is the judge, as described earlier. With me, she respected analysis once again. Remembered that as a girl when she was deprived of something, a girl not letting her play with a doll, her attitude was, this does not affect me.

Discussion

Growing up, she wanted to be a man and not a woman. The presence of breasts was a minus, an absence, a sign of a loss in the gaze of the Other. More than as an *objet a* that covers a hole, the breast was the signifier of the minus phi, of the lack, of not having the phallus. This meaning of wounding loss was further emphasized by the disgust toward bleeding from her genitals in menstruation.

She found her first husband threatening. His erect penis was feared and wounding. Although he was quite a catch for her, she found his demand to be recognized as a master, annoying and demeaning. In Hegelian fashion, the master needs a servant to recognize them as a master; the slavery of the master and the mastery of the servant are revealed at the end of their relationship, which leaves her with remorse for having destroyed him.

T wanted to be a man or a superwoman but not the woman as the signifier of symbolic castration, of the lack in the Other. To be a professional woman, she did not need to be a man because she was encouraged to study by both parents and mother was already a successful academic. In her mind, a woman corresponded to being a wife and a mother but not at the exclusion of being a professional woman or an intellectual. This is the place where she refuses symbolic castration and sexual difference under the fear of the imaginary father/phallus experienced as an imaginary form of castration as in the example of having breasts, menstruation, and children. Having means not having.

The disavowed symbolic femininity returns in the Imaginary and the Real. In the Real of jouissance, she is always having to be a servant to other women, and she fears she will end up being the hyper-servant of the grotesque and uncanny daughter she did not want. In the Imaginary, she enjoys being of service and a sexual servant of many men so long as she is not limited to serving only one man. If her partner is of service to her or his daughter, this causes her to look elsewhere for the man who may have another woman instead of serving her. The service of the man is seen as an imaginary form of castration. The service of the man means both the man serving her and her serving the man.

Her desire is for the desire of the mother. This is the mother of the Imaginary and not of the Symbolic mother. The maternal gift is not absent. The mother makes herself absent as a mother in the sense that she desires things beyond the child but remains in a position of omnipotence. Such omnipotence is limited by the imaginary father but not in the sense of the idealized father but in the sense of the brutal father (yells, farts, and makes arbitrary demands at times) and of the father who desires and gives satisfaction to the mother. The mother enjoyed sex with the father, and in fact, it was so good that she felt that this enjoyment enslaved her to him because otherwise she would have left him. But there is no imaginary idealized father or the ideal of a symbolic father sustained by the emptiness of the function. This is directly related to the metaphor of the father in the mother's speech. The mother appears as omnipotent and the father as a burden. T stays in the position of identification with and being the cause of the mother's desire. Her desire is not completely displaced in the direction of finding and avowing the law of the father that then could lead to an idealization of the father and then to a falling off from this idealization. Her phantasm fills the lack in the Other in that she identifies with the omnipotent mother and searches for the idealized non-lacking father which defends against the presence of femininity which could serve as a guarantor of the emptiness of the symbolic phallus function.

The mother does not take care of the father; the father wants to leave because the mother is fat.

What she thinks of herself	*What the other thinks of her*
Here she does not know what to say. Perhaps give a class that nobody has given before.	Female students say that gives the best class. This is what she is capable of doing with her body.
She constantly loses her thesis.	In Mexico the old men of academia don't like her.
She cannot have the symbolic phallus.	

The construction of femininity: The spectacle of my body and its potency. The gaze of mothers. In the dance everything goes and then it ends. I am the dream of my mother, her with her polio and her fat body. Father is sinful and agile, and a good lover. The competition with males began at home. Weaning, and rejection, the perception of weakness, the ideal of masculinity the competition with my brothers.

In her case, she had anxiety but was not high; otherwise, she was not symptomatic. So, we will give her a −2 for anxiety and grief as an expression of the perceived lack of femininity. Because she had a high level of education, we also gave her a 3i. Her capacity for analysis allows her to change. She met these objectives at the end of the personal analysis and went from −2i to 2i and from 3i to 5i.

In the case of another analysand, he had a dream that provides a good example of the agalma. He was in a synagogue with altar in Jerusalem. I was the rabbi/teacher. He opens a secret box that has a cardboard with Hebrew letters. The letters have extreme power, although he does not know what they mean. In the next scene, he is holding a stone called the tiger's eye. He wants to tell me he is leaving and asks me what the letters mean. I tell him it is the name of my grandfather, Levi Yitzchak, who meditated on his own name. He wants to smuggle the rock back into the US; he flirts with my wife and becomes afraid that Arabs may stab him.

At first, the agalma appears in its entire splendor: the holy and awesome setting, the sense of spiritual delight and the mysterious, the signifiers of the symbolic father, and the precious stone or jewel. The phallic and narcissistic significance of the agalma is only secondarily revealed when the letters without a fixed signification become the letters that he attributed to the name of my grandfather, who was supposed to have used them to meditate on his own name. For Jews, this would be a heretical act given that Jews only meditate on the Tetragrammaton (the four-lettered name of G-d), the meaning of which remains unknown. In addition, the reference to my grandfather meditating on his own name was linked by association to the fact that this analysand engaged in a ritual act of performing fellatio on himself. The alleged name of his grandfather stands as a signifier of the imaginary father/phallus. He then tries to steal (smuggle) the imaginary phallus and use it to flirt with his wife. The aggressive nature of the act is revealed by the projective or paranoid fear of Arabs.

Socrates professed no knowledge except that of his own not knowing. He believed that people know both less and more than what they think they do. To those who appeared to know, he showed them that they actually did not know, and to those who appeared not to know, he showed them that in fact they did know: 'This object that you apparently want from me and that you think I have, is your own object. Not that you have it or are it, but "it" lives in you, as your own fantasy.' Lacan compared Socrates's response to the subjective position of the analyst or to what Lacan called the desire of the analyst.

An analysand had a vision; it was the evening of his wedding in 1985. Suddenly he spontaneously entered in a state of bliss that me knew from the earlier experience of circumcision. Then the space around him disappeared, and he was in empty space; in front of me, marble stairway appeared, leading up to a platform where an old man with a long beard dressed in a white robe stood in a very equanimous state. Most strikingly behind him was a full moon shining like the sun.

From there, he went to the place where the wedding was going to take place, and upon entering, he encountered a lay rabbi who looked just like the old man on the platform.

The second vision was when he went to Israel. At the beginning of Shabbat HaGadol, he walked down to the Temple in Jerusalem. Shabbat HaGadol is a sabbath of consolation, after the 11th of Av when the second temple was destroyed. He was born on the 9th of Av or July 30. As he approached the Wailing Wall, his mind went into a state of deep bliss and radiance, and when he looked up the wall at the top and the meeting place of the wall and heaven, he saw the same full moon shining like the sun.

In a third vision, he was the retreat director at the Berkeley Zen Center, sitting in the front seat. In the afternoon, during an open period of meditation, the sesshin director also sat facing the wall, rather than sitting facing the community of practitioners. Against the wall appeared the full moon shining like the sun with two Hindu figures by the side engaged in a sacred dance. The G-d of enlightenment, or brightness according to the Kabbalah, is both Jewish and Hindu, according to his visions. Hinduism historically came before Judaism, although it may come after Abraham as described in the Bible.

The sun is the source of light not only as an object but also as a condensation of energy present in all things. The sun shining like the moon is also a metaphor of inner subjective and mental life.

He struggled a lot about conflicting relative loyalties to Zen Buddhism and Judaism, whether he needed to decide between one or the other, conflicts with his wife over this, and the issues of identity that this brought up. He felt very drawn to Judaism, because of the spirituality mentioned earlier, but felt that these Jewish experiences were influenced and made possible by Zen experience that he was not ready to give up.

A lot of other Jews did not seem to be having these experiences. At one point, after he returned from a trip to Israel, he went back to the Zen center, and before going in, he asked Buddha in heaven for a very clear sign that Zen practice was for him and that he should stay with it. If he did not get this sign, he was prepared to abandon the practice. Once he took a seat in the Zendo, or meditation hall, he entered a very deep samadhi (an experience that has preceded all of the visionary and deep spiritual experiences he has had) or state of calm, luminous concentration and bliss, and then somehow, he found himself up in the air in the middle of the room with Mel and their bodies, in the lotus posture, went right through one another in absolute transparency. This was an experiential realization of the teaching of interdependence. Their bodies fused and passed through each other without obstacle. It was interesting that this was an instance during which a supplicative prayer to the Jewish absolute did work, yet he received a Buddhist response to the prayer from a Jewish Zen teacher. So 'who' was listening? It was 'Juda Buddha', the Tathagata.

Low-Heeled Shoes as a Mark of Femininity

This is a woman in her late 30s, who just finished four years of analysis on online video, occasional phone sessions at times, with office sessions once at the beginning of the analysis and then another set of sessions in the middle phase of the analysis. The analysis ended online.

Half of my work at this point is online or on the phone; the other half is in the office. I work with people in different parts of the country and in different countries, mostly in English. I began working online once I became a control analyst 11 years ago. I worked as a psychologist/psychotherapist for 10 years and then as an analyst in formation for about 7 years, all in the office. I had worked as a supervisor for decades before that and as director of training in a large psychiatric clinic.

In the office, the analysand enters the office and lies down on the couch with the analyst behind them. If the patient prefers, the analysis can begin face-to-face at first during the preliminary sessions until they decide to work together.

Online, we meet via videoconference, and at first, if there is any business, it is okay to start face-to-face in the office or online.

Once the analysand lies down, the analyst is at the computer behind the couch. Or, if this is not possible, the analysand lies down with their feet resting on an Ottoman chair, if not a couch, and then turns off their video. Analysis can also be done over the phone.

For this case presentation, the initial presentation of symptoms was vague, and it was unclear what she wanted to keep, what she wanted to change, and if her jouissance was pleasure or suffering. Symptoms and fantasies emerged in the analysis over time, and they were embedded in her character traits.

Character traits are usually in the body: a stiff upper lip, a nervous gesture, or copying somebody else's style of speaking.

Character traits are either egosyntonic or egodystonic. *Egodystonic* means that problems are problems for others but not for the ego. The ego loves its traits that are a problem for others.

Symptoms, rather than character traits, are always egodystonic because they cause pain for the subject.

Symptoms

1. 'Anxiety is stirred up in the core of my being' with respect to a man she was seeing briefly when she began the analysis. 'I just want to be close to him, to ravish him, to make him love me'.

   I must warn you that I use the foul language the analysand used. Analysts have to use this language, not only because it contains lalangue (language of the unconscious – for example, 'motherfucker') but because we are like medical doctors who need to work with the body without standards of proper social speech getting in the way.

   'I know that fucking someone the way I fucked him isn't the way girls get boys to love them'. She rejects passive femininity.

2. She said that her relationship with her father did not provide sustenance and was harmful.

   It was difficult for her to imagine herself in a long-term relationship. The first sexual difference is with the father and then in latency is transferred to other boys, and in puberty, it becomes sexual.

   'The closest was thinking of buying a duplex with me living next door to the person, something that could point to something lasting, but it never played itself out'.
3. She gets angry and jealous in relationships. She thought he was interested in other women. She had an elaborate fantasy with a friend of his. He never met her; he lived in Los Angeles, and nothing was going on between them. She feared losing him to another woman. It had something to do with going back to using drugs.

   She has a history of drug use since she ran away from home at age 12 and dropped out of school. She prostituted herself a few times to obtain drugs and spent a total of 5 years in prison due to stealing and committing fraud to obtain drugs.

   She became sober through Narcotics Anonymous and was already sober when she started her analysis. She finished high school and college in prison and was in a PhD program in women's studies when she started her analysis, was dissatisfied with North American gender studies, and came looking for Lacanian psychoanalysis, which is a slowly but surely growing trend in the United States.
4. She is so malleable and has no identity,

   She became what everyone around her was and she idealized men and fetishized them. She resists white middle-class shit in the university. She idealized street credibility

   She rejects trashy and respectability. She occupies a space in the middle and does not fit in in either place. She does not know what identity she wants to affirm.

   Lacan said the woman does not exist in the Symbolic only 'ex-sists' in the Real, so she has the flexibility or the disorientation to be an Other woman or the ideal woman.

Family History

Her parents had her when they were 18 and were not married. Her mother's family did not like her father, who was bright and handsome but a recluse and antisocial, fitting a character type not uncommon in the US known as a survivalist. Poor whites are retreating into the woods to survive the onslaught of what they perceive as minorities and blacks taking over the country. Rich liberal whites have 'integrated' minorities into the market, but poor whites have been forsaken and remain the archenemies of both.

She was raised by her maternal grandparents until age 8 when her grandfather died, and this was a major cataclysm for her, not only because she had been the apple of her grandfather's eye but because she then went to live with her parents. Up until then, her mother was like a sister who came to visit and was fun to play with.

She lived with her mother first in a trailer park. Her mother was using drugs and alcohol and had different lovers; she ran away to her father's house. Her father lived with no plumbing, electricity, or hot water, with only an outhouse for a bathroom.

Her father would try to discipline her in rather crude ways, telling her she was stupid and trying to enforce gender roles. This problem had a prior history where we see the emergence of the *objet a*. With her grandparents, her grandmother was in charge of discipline, and the grandfather was the loving 'grandmotherly' type in her eyes. Her grandmother caught her peeing standing up repeatedly as her favorite form and insisted that she had to pee sitting down as girls do. She also liked to wear men's underwear and men's shoes, almost military boots. The father continued with this, and in addition, he told her that she was a woman and explained how men and women have sex and that she had a vagina and men would put their penis inside her. So she hated penetration, which she experienced as getting fucked over. Her urinary flow was her favorite object (tells jokes), and she disliked her vagina, which she identified with the total body of her mother, whom she regarded as ugly, fat, smelly white trash.

Her favorite form of sex was anal sex, and she liked to penetrate both sexes anally as well as receive anal penetration. From the back or anally, there is no sexual difference.

Let me quote you some of her speech:

> As soon as I see him, I know I'll do dirty things to him. We make out in public and then go back to his place where I proceed to ravish him. No one has ever eaten out his asshole. He loves it and is terrified. I know the way I'm touching him is the way that men are supposed to touch women, and I know, because I know, that men say they want this, like this, and then, faced with it, they don't. But I can't help myself. I can't be someone else. Not now, not here. I just want to consume his body, him. He tells me he's never been with someone like me. Like what? I ask. Like a real woman, he tells me. What does that mean? I ask. Someone who knows what she wants, who does what she wants. In almost the same breath, he tells me that he's supposed to be the man, that I'm being the man, that he feels like a girl. It comes up again and again. The way I eat his asshole is like the way he eats pussy. The way he moans is the way he makes women moan when it does that to them. I find all of this incredibly sexy and he finds it terrifying. Terrifying, exciting, pleasurable, but terrifying, maybe painful. Enjoyable?

> Even though this is sex for me, with no future in sight, no commitment, there is still something so serious about it, something so not-casual, despite the circumstances. I could never do this with more than one person at a time. I'm giving him too much of myself. I give too much of myself when I do this.

We say that men conflate sex and love and that women know, on the contrary, that love is in language, discourse, and speech. That is why women have to talk so much about sex and love and men do not.

> These things I do with my body, with my mouth and my hands, they say something, but they seem to say something that I can't say in language. The sexual drive in the Real is outside language.
>
> I've been thinking about the lover she had when she started analysis and about his withdrawal, wondering, again, why I do this to myself. He says it's work that is keeping him away, but I'm sure it's not. I'm also not sure, which is what makes things so difficult. I hate not knowing.

Then she met her current boyfriend. Before meeting him, she was fantasizing about planning her future to live with a girlfriend who was also bisexual and androgynous because she did not believe in commitments or long-term relationships or commitments with men, something she considered stupid and conventional.

Her current boyfriend broke up with girlfriend, and she was not that into him.

She likes him but is not symptomatic (laughs). She knows who she is and does not want to be seen with him; he is balding, dorky, and nerdy; he feels inferior to her; she is critical and smarter than him; and she knows what she is talking about and has her shit together. She sees herself as a 'whole' person. 'Whole' here is a euphemism. She ends up being confrontational because he is boring and does not self-reflect. 'What is the less favorite thing about me? I don't do relationships; you won't lock me down'.

'I like him, but I don't feel overly liking him. He is not annoying. She is neither in love nor annoyed. Neither of those ways. It's nice, fine'. Then she asked him, 'Do you want to come to my parents for Xmas?'

'I like my mother seeing me be normal or in a relationship. She is seeing me with boyfriend in a way that does not correspond with my reality. Mother's apprehension of the relationship matters'.

She says that her relationship with men fall into two categories: felt rejected and humiliated more like her father versus men who spoil her like her grandfather. She stalks men who are like her grandfather: 'They look dorky, not cool, disgusting, I could do better than him'. She is embarrassed. The bad boy, haughty, asshole – she likes to conquer them, more like her dad. What they have that she wants that gets displaced into being bad asshole. Other types are the tattooed, cool, and married. Someone she should be seen with. Her boyfriend is damaged, aloof, unavailable.

She thinks that she is better than her boyfriend: cooler, smarter, better looking, a come-up for him; he knows that. 'Don't you feel better about yourself now that I desire you'. She does not feel a need for him. With the other men, she cannot get her hands off them. When she is sucking dick and eat their assholes, she sees herself degrading herself.

'I am too good to be doing these things with somebody like Grandfather.' She feels conflicted because he is a good person. She is enjoying having sex with her boyfriend. She loves rubbing and sucking dick. She should not do it because he is not good enough. It is pretty knotty, naughty. Dirty, slutty. She had a dream that she was in a football game, responsible for the balls, and scores a touchdown; then she was called by her name.

Associations: likes watching football, brings out violence. Does not like her name. Mom wanted to name her Elizabeth. C-section. Hard labor. Her father named her while her mother had 24 hours of labor.

She does not know why her name. Her mother still calls her Elizabeth. She remembers hating her name at age 11. She does not feel like a man or woman. She does not like either name.

She does not like the way they sound. Her first name is harsh. She hates her last name. With her cats, she refers to herself in the third person. Her name is a common name. Her father's grandmother and his sister have that name.

She is in charge of the balls and scores a touchdown. She does not like cheerleaders. She would have preferred an androgynous name used by both men and women. It is a rejection of the father.

In a dream, she is preparing to get raped. A guy gives her lubricant and says this big brutal guy will come in and rape her and hurt her with a big penis. She prepares herself for rape, prepares herself for the pain. She starts masturbating so she is loose and wet.

Associations

Fantasy about a big guy. Fat and muscular. He tattoos her, and she gets turned on with the pressing on her body. She is the sexy one, is or has the phallus, and they are weak and disgusting and subordinate. They give her head. Or she is nothing and they are a big penis using her as a sexual object. Or she identifies with the big fat penis or imaginary phallus, and she is the one raping a guy in the ass. Or she masturbates to porn where she is both the woman getting raped and the man doing the raping.

Heterosexual intercourse is either women getting raped by men treated as a sexual object, which she does not enjoy intercourse, or she masturbates to porn in which women are getting raped, and she gives herself her own orgasm. She could only have a clitorial orgasm and only if she stimulated herself during sex.

Her current boyfriend, to whom she became quite attached and developed a desire for a long-term relationship with him, did not like anal sex and did not want to be penetrated, resulting in a loss of jouissance for her, but the relationship became more important, and she had to come to terms with the lack of sexual rapport. She came to enjoy vaginal sex, although the jouissance was not as intense, and she let him stimulate her clitoris although she preferred to do it herself and so did he.

Anorexic Symptom

She is a ribbon in a dream, her fragmented body turning small, floating away, disappearing, being chased after by a man. 'I have starved myself. I can feel it in my body, my electrolytes off, my head in a vice, on the verge of losing consciousness when I stand up. But I'm not really losing weight. I'm still a cow. Maybe'.

She reported this initially in relationship to a dream but then never brought it again and did not seem to have a problem with it or with her weight. Then she went to Korea, attended a conference on anorexia, and began talking about it.

Despite her identification with masculinity, she said she idealized petite hyperfeminine and submissive women. She admired and rejected the stereotypically feminine women: 'I can't be it and don't want to be it'. She has a perceived lack of femininity within herself that she idealizes in the Other and at the same time rejects for herself.

She began starving herself and losing weight, and she looked emaciated and had a cadaveric face like a concentration camp survivor. She did not report it as a problem and resisted seeing it as such. I focused on her interest in anorexia and going to a conference. She acknowledged always touching her bones, a protruding bone. I had her associate to the protruding bone, and she came up with a boner as a metaphor for imaginary phallus. I tell her this is a woman's way to be a man.

She was losing awareness of crossing the line into death. She enjoyed it; it was a high, her anorexic jouissance for the nothing. I expressed concern about the risk that this could lead her to death. As a result of my concern, she began weighing herself and established a limit for her weight despite the deadly enjoyment.

Shoes

Eventually she disclosed that despite her preference for men's shoes, she had five trunks full of women's shoes. She was not satisfied with men's shoes and had a desire for women's shoes but could not wear them and was not comfortable in them; they felt like a simulacrum rather than a masquerade. We remember that *Oedipus* in Greek means 'swollen foot'. I told her that she was trying to discover what a woman is and that neither a man nor the simulacrum of a woman satisfied the question and suggested that she could leave it undefined and empty and merely in the form of a question without an answer. (For the record, *swollen* in Sanskrit means 'empty', therefore the emptiness of Oedipus.) She was happy with this and began using a feminine version of basketball shoes now made trendy for women as well as flats with flat or low heels.

Termination

She finished her dissertation and her PhD but lost her insurance and could not afford the fee by herself. She was able to get a job as an academic, something that is not easy in the US, to say the least, but that does not start for another six months. We observe here the relationship between the traversal of the fantasy or the fall of the *objet a* and the changes in love and work that Freud considered sufficient criteria for the aim/end of the analysis.

I subjectively would have preferred for the analysis to end once her professional practice as an academic was consolidated. But in fact, Lacan says the analyst ends the session but the analysand ends the analysis. Now she is a disciple of her symptom, and the work with the sinthome continues post-termination and has post-termination effects. She had enough of me and the analysis, and I agreed.

The analysis was difficult for her because her symptoms were lodged in character traits that were egosyntonic. I systematically always explored the symptoms in relationship to her character traits, and this was not pleasant for her, but she stuck to it. She bore what was unbearable about analysis. I systematically never gave her any room to regard her symptoms as a problem for me but not for her, with the exception perhaps of the risk of death due to anorexia. In analysis, you cannot analyze a symptom, as a psychoanalytic symptom, without first clarifying the subjective position in relationship to the symptom as a form of jouissance. We never take for granted that the symptom is a problem, however painful, although we at first strategically pretend this to be the case. We tacitly know that the analysand is in love with their symptoms and the symptom is how the analysand 'makes out' with the Unconscious, as Lacan says in RSI.

Because the analysis was painful, or open-heart surgery, she never expressed much regret for losing me. I decided to make a mistake on purpose, following what Harari taught me that an analyst is established by their mistakes in the Freudian sense of parapraxis. I simply said once that I would miss our work together so that I would remain as a pure desire and an acceptance of lack, no longer an imaginary object, whether idealized or persecutory, and an object that she could discard. It was true, however, and not make-believe; otherwise, I would not have said it.

Conclusion

Are there any structured signifiers that are universal or common to most people? This is what Freud's biographer, Ernest Jones (1916), argued. Here, Lacanian signifiers are equivalent to Jungian archetypes. Archetypes, for Jung, although images, were symbolic elements equivalent to genes.

The signifiers for the cases were virgin, gigolo, hole, staff, symbols, castration, phallic woman, authority, father, big Other, son, mother, doctor, sinner, man, 'fucker', snake, parricide, bohemian, woman, sinner, girl as a scholar, feminine jouissance, mystic jouissance, peachy, little devil, special boy, fallen angel, and mystical jouissance.

The signifiers are the Real pieces that fell off the structure and that operate in reality, rather than the other way around. It is not that the structure operates in reality and the pieces fall away into oblivion. The structure is invisible and does not operate in reality; only the Real pieces do.

What do I mean by 'Real structure'? I refer to the oedipal structure that is no longer Symbolic, as Lacan said. Lacan said that the Oedipus complex was a dream of Freud and, I would add, represents a mathematical structure. Oedipus is Real as a mathematical structure and virtual as a dream, or fiction. The pure mother is a virgin; the obedient boy could be used as a gigolo by sacred or secular authorities. He contains the hole of the vagina in the anus. The mother represents the lack of the Other. The complete mother is the phallic mother who has the pants in the house. Now she can wear the pants either because she stole the pants from the father or because the father gave them to her.

The father represents the values of the culture and ancestors. The doctor is holy, like women, while men are sinners and fornicators/*masterbators*. Are girls undisciplined, as Freud said, 'They have no superego', or are girls more disciplined in school? In any case, a scholar girl is something special, and if you are special enough, you will find her in a library lane riding a white pony and selecting her favorite books. The girl in the white pony is Athena emerging from inside her father's head or, at least, from the bosom of his storehouse memory.

Are children pure or perverse? Children have no fixed ego, so they are not perverse. There is no difference between a child's purity and the mystic jouissance of the beginner's mind. The end is like the beginning, and after having gone through the childishness and horror of unconscious fantasy and polymorphous perversion, the analysand goes back to being a child with mature and wise characteristics.

The capacity for sublimation is a drive that I measure with imaginary numbers. One can also acquire higher levels of sublimation ascending the *y*- (i) imaginary axis. The lessening of symptoms increases the potential for sublimation, making more energy available for other uses. However, I acknowledge that assessing the capacity for sublimation is an intuitive and conceptual axiom that does not have to be proven in science. It depends on interests, capacities, and creative activities. However, a more precise instrument could also be developed.

To conclude, I offer a table of the signifiers shared by all subjects in this book. This is not a representative sample in the statistical sense but a representative sample of norms established not by statistics but by normative society. I note that anxiety is a more common symptom than depression. I can conclude that the hypothesis advanced by many is true. The 21st century is a century not of depression but of anxiety, the result of 'too much' rather than not enough: encore. The 20th century was the century of two World Wars: impermanence, death, and loss.

Case of M	Martin	Chinese	S	Literary Benevolence	Case of J
Failure of identification with father	Desire to kill father	Refusal of father	My son the doctor	My son the brilliant scholar	His phallus is the name of his kabbalistic father in the transference
Special to mother	Special to mother	Special to mother	Special to mother	Special to mother	
Anxiety depersonalization		anxiety addiction	anxiety irritability	anxiety depression	Anxiety grief
Case of M		Martin	Chinese	S	Literary Benevolence
Failure of identification with father		Desire to kill father	Refusal of father	My son the doctor	My son the brilliant scholar
Special to mother		Special to mother	Special to mother	Special to mother	Special to mother
Anxiety depersonalization		anxiety addiction		anxiety irritability	anxiety depression

A positive response to treatment is represented by a decrease of x numbers and an increase of i numbers. Higher levels of sublimation predict better outcomes, and the capacity for sublimation can be increased in a virtuous cycle (indicated by prime numbers). Sublimation is not a socialized ego drive but an evolved form of jouissance. The ego is useful as a concept to understand narcissism. The reality principle is a principle of the subject. The concept of self can be used for either undifferentiated or recognizable self-experience.

Finally, if we plot all the complex numbers on a complex plane, we find that posttreatment all the numbers are on the right-side imaginary side of the graph. How do we obtain imaginary complex numbers that are both golden and imaginary? And how does this relate to the question of the phallus, which for Lacan was equivalent to the golden number, and how does the golden number 1.684 (a symbolic phallus:$\Phi \rightarrow -\left(\sqrt{1}\right)$ in a quadratic equation transforms into an imaginary number and a different form of jouissance? Phi transforms into i or (√−1). The 1.68 includes infinitesimals, while the imaginary number is a negative unit that cannot be subdivided further.

> Mathematically Phi – phi (1,618 − 0,618) = 1. This can be seen as the formula for the phallic function of castration. Phi – phi = the 'symbolic phallus' minus the 'imaginary phallus' . . . −phi or the lack of the imaginary phallus generates a lack-of-being; a hole within the whole that subjects endlessly try to fill with objets a. It does not work because −phi is a signifier without a signified (phallic function). It is a symbolic castration that creates a gap thereby representing a point of lack in the subject.
>
> (Moncayo and Romanowicz, 2015, p. 130)

Phi − phi = 1 is the formula for symbolic castration, where only by accepting the lack (−phi) with the help of Phi can the subject arrive at One as an imaginary number or i (imaginary in the mathematical, not Lacanian, sense). Otherwise, the subject keeps looking for the fantasy object in reality and in the axis of real numbers (real in the mathematical sense and in the sense of external reality).

According to the formula Phi − phi, as the formula for symbolic castration, Phi subtracts the a (phi) and turns every i(a) and i (a′1,2,3,4) into a 1 that can be used as either a real or imaginary number. Phi is the quantity or power by which phi changes into 1 as either a series of real numbers or a series of imaginary numbers. In this sense, the formula for castration also qualifies as a logarithm for images.

By phi missing from Phi, Phi becomes either a real 1 or an imaginary 1. One has the *objet a* missing from it. With a or −a missing in real whole-body images, the subject tries to fill the hole with other alter egos and their missing *objet a* in a futile exercise that is played at the level of images. Instead of another whole image or number, what needs to be symbolized and made manifest in numbers is the 1 as an imaginary number that appears in the hole in the image. Otherwise, the alleged whole objects and alter egos or intersubjective others go from being whole numbers to being like the song of Ricky Martin: 'a little bit of Monica, Gloria, and Veronica in my life,' the partial *objet a* of the subject in its various iterations.

Plotnitsky (2009) has quoted Leibniz in this regard: 'Imaginary roots are a subtle and wonderful resort of the divine spirit, a kind of hermaphrodite between existence and non-existence (inter En and non Ens Amphibio)'.

> [T]he square root of −1 does not correspond to anything that is subject to our intuition, anything real-in the mathematical sense of the term – and yet it must be conserved, along with its full functioning.
>
> (Lacan, 1959, p. 29)

The phallus is a missing or non-existing object/signifier and a signifier without a signified (Ø) and in this sense bears a resemblance to the existence/nonexistence of imaginary numbers as well as to the mark of the unmarked.

The bracket on the zero is 1 but leaves the zero intact as a concept and a number. The bar instead makes the zero a no concept, a no number, a no name, and an empty space.

Within Lacanian psychoanalysis, the barred zero is a pure form of the negative that is not a point in space in the sense of an object but simply a symbolic empty place of substitution and movement for representations. It is in this sense that Lacan says that the symbolic phallus appears in the place of the signifier of a lack or the lack of a signifier. This is even though the symbolic phallus as Capital Phi is also a golden number within the axis of real numbers.

Within the symbolic function of Capital Phi, small +phi and −phi represent the presence and absence of substitutive and imaginary signifiers for the phallus. But why then does Lacan use the square root of −1 as a signifier for the phallus that is an imaginary number and not a real number like the golden number?

$\sqrt{-1}$ is an impossible number: there is no square root of −1. Yet we are using it in calculations in mathematics and physics all the time. In the same way, although the phallus as such may not exist (impossible to represent), it may also lead to true conclusions regarding certain forms of phenomena described by psychoanalysis.

Imaginary numbers may be considered impossible, yet they follow all the basic rules of mathematics like addition, subtraction, and multiplication. In addition, the unit imaginary number, i, has the property of cycling through four different values of multiplication, as shown:

$$i^1 = i$$
$$i^2 = -1$$
$$i^3 = -i$$
$$i^4 = 1$$

$$i^5 = i \times i^4 = i$$
$$i^6 = i^2 \times i^4 = -i$$
$$i^7 = i^3 \times i^4 = -i$$
$$i^8 = i^4 \times i^4 = 1$$

The cycling of i yields four terms: i, −1, −i, and 1.

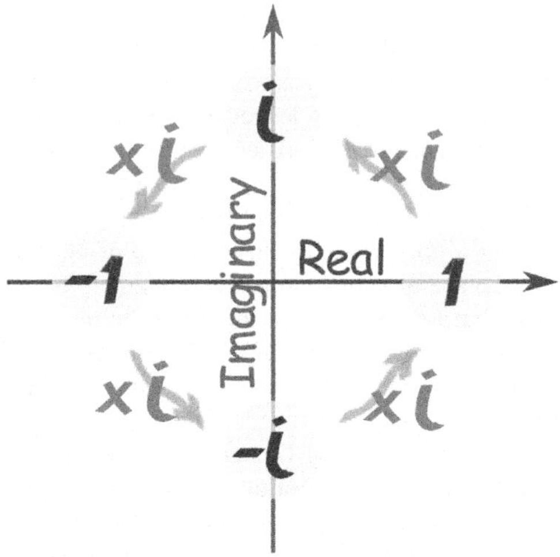

The neutral point between 1 and −1 and i and −i represents the center of two axes: the imaginary and the real axes. The Imaginary can be the fantasy of the imagination (archetype), rather than the Imaginary. For example, the Nazis used the swastika symbol of Buddhist origins and perverted it with an imaginary meaning. The imagination is based on the poetics of metaphor and resemblance and reveals the glory of emptiness, the consummated nature. The real axis is never Real. It consists of our drives and fixations that need to be sublated not by the Imaginary but by the imagination.

In the graph, there is a circle that combines both axes: I, −1, −i, 1. From this circle, we can extend a wave of water, or a target, for example, to 2i, −2, −2i, 2, 2i, and so on. This represents Buddhism as a series of circles within circles, with the teaching representing the particles and the waves representing the experience of jouissance/meditation.

I can understand numbers as quantum particles and not only as numbers that are part of a symbolic system laid on top of ontology and the Real of the things themselves. Instead, imaginary numbers are the things in themselves as particles, not as waves as waves numbers remain outside the symbolic system. The Real is a series of quantum waves in the emptiness of the vacuum that are perceived as the forms of matter (the visual world is a simulation).

Quantum waves are Real energy outside the Symbolic system that is measured with nontrivial zeros in the 0.5 critical line. You have waves starting at zero and expanding outward to 2 to 4 with phase space-time being the space in-between diacritical numbers indicated by the arrows $0 \rightarrow 2 \rightarrow 4 \rightarrow$ etc. We can visualize how the waves irradiate from a point 0 that does not exist: 0, 1, 2, 3, and so on.

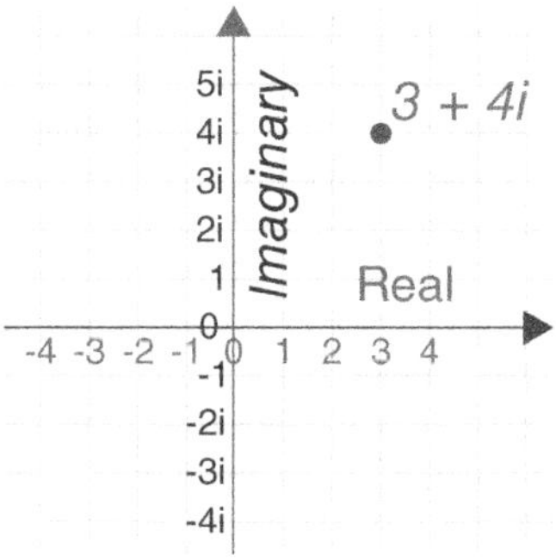

https://www.mathsisfun.com/algebra/complex-plane.html
accessed March 5, 2023.

Before we proceed further, we need to clarify certain similarities and differences between mathematical and Lacanian terms. The use of imaginary numbers in mathematics differs from the concept of the Imaginary in Lacan. Images in the sense of the Imaginary have no diacritical numbers unless we reduce color to number. For this reason, imaginary numbers in a Lacanian sense are Symbolic. By the same reasoning, real numbers in the mathematical sense are not Real in the Lacanian use of the term.

Lacan talks about the phallus in several ways throughout his work:

1. Lacan writes about the imaginary phallus as 1 and −1 in real axis.
2. He also speaks about the imaginary phallus and the *objet a* in terms of the golden number proportion 0.618.
3. The phallus is also described as i number ($\sqrt{-1}$).

Using 1 and −1 is a very crude way of talking about the phallus as animal imaginary genital jouissance without signifiers. With speaking beings and language, phi and −phi depend on castration that assigns them their place.

Lacan said that the null set or the signifier of a symbolic lack is related to the Capital Phi or the symbolic phallus, which is an absence and is equivalent to symbolic castration and does not have the positive and negative signs that Lacan ascribes to the imaginary phallus as phi and −phi. It is the symbolic phallus that gives access to phallic jouissance. Without castration, there is no phallic jouissance, properly speaking; there may be copulation or rape but no phallic jouissance.

But ultimately, the phallus does not exist, and to experience this void, or the phallus that does not exist as the no signified, may be traumatic.

The subject needs the name as the symbolic phallus (Phi) that substitutes for the imaginary phallus (−phi). Then from the name that is meaningless or is a “no name” or simply “this” the experience of the void as the Other jouissance is possible.

Lacan says that a name brings a relative stop to the sliding of signifiers and to the production of a new imaginary *objet a*. But the signifier of a lack in the Other is the name of the nameless or is the name that points to an absence that is also a presence in the Real. This is where the name also links to the Real face of the *objet a* as the index of a void of presence and an Other jouissance not-all under the phallic function, for which feminine jouissance is one of its forms. This is what the square root of −1 represents, in our opinion.

The symbolic phallus moves the subject in the direction of the square root of −1 because it does not exist and has no direct reference to the penis. In 1973, Lacan stated that the symbolic phallus is 'the signifier which does not have a signified' (Seminar XX, 1972–1973, p. 75). The square root of −1 is a special signifier without a signified or better a number without a number.

The statement that the symbolic phallus or F appears in the place of the lack of the signifier in the Other, seems to link the F and the lack in the Other, the symbol of which is the same symbol as the null or empty set (Ø). Lacan uses the math symbol for the null set for the signifier of a lack in the Other.

$\emptyset \rightarrow \Phi \rightarrow \sqrt{-1}$ (Formula adapted by Miller, 2015)

The lack in the Other (Ø) transforms into Phi (Φ) and into $\sqrt{-1}$. The $\sqrt{-1}$ is outside phallic jouissance. The missing signifier transforms into a structure with a missing piece that transforms into symbolic wholeness in emptiness (a unary negation). The law and the structure do not exist or dissipate, yet they generate the order of the structure. The law is ultimately the Law of Wu as a unary negation. The mystery is how the law of emptiness (Kong) transforms into the Taoist and Confucian virtues of particularity and propriety.

$$(\Phi \rightarrow -\surd -1)$$

$$(-\surd -1 \rightarrow \Phi)$$

Phallic jouissance can go beyond phallic jouissance and become the third jouissance, the third jouissance can go back to the second, and the second go back to the first. Mathematically, Phi − phi (1.618 − 0.618) = 1. This can be seen as the formula for the phallic function of castration. Phi – phi = the 'symbolic phallus' minus the 'imaginary phallus'. The first jouissance represents the bad infinity of metonymy and displacement of representations.

Negative phi or the lack of the imaginary phallus generates a lack-of-being, a hole within the whole that subjects endlessly try to fill with *objet a*. It does not work because −phi is a signifier without signified (phallic function). It is a symbolic castration that creates a gap, thereby representing a point of lack in the subject.

A positive response to treatment is represented by a decrease of *x* numbers and an increase in the *y*-axis, or i numbers. Higher levels of sublimation predict better outcomes, and the capacity for sublimation can be increased in a virtuous cycle (indicated by prime numbers)' (above) and at the same time the sublime number ($\sqrt{-1}$) goes back into phallic jouissance. The sublime number refers to the quantification of events: art, religion, scholarship, exercise, martial culture, music, and the like.

Cases also retain numbers on the bottom-right quadrant of imaginary numbers. This means that the tree of knowledge not only ascends to the heights but also descends with deep roots inside the earth. In a case with a history of addiction, the subject remains prone to addiction within sobriety. This means that the subject remains prone to speak of the Real without words, or with mathematics. These are the numbers in a binary matrix that represent the character and analysis of the subject.

1. Chinese Unconscious

$$\begin{pmatrix} 2 & -2i \\ 2i & 2 \end{pmatrix}$$

$$(2+-2\text{i})\times(2\text{i}+2)(4+4\text{i})$$

2. Case of S

$$\begin{pmatrix} 1 & -2i \\ 2i & 1 \end{pmatrix}$$

$$(1+-2\text{i})\times(2\text{i}+1)(2+4\text{i})$$

3. Case of Martin

$$\begin{pmatrix} 3 & -2i \\ -2i & 3 \end{pmatrix}$$

$$(3+-2\text{i})\times(-2\text{i}+3)\rightarrow(6+-4\text{i})$$

$$\begin{pmatrix} 2 & -5i \\ -5i & 2 \end{pmatrix}$$

$$(2+-5\text{i})\times(-5\text{i}+2)\rightarrow 4+10\text{i})$$

4. Literary Benevolence

$$\begin{pmatrix} 0 & -7i \\ -7i & 0 \end{pmatrix}$$

$$(0+-7)\times(-7+0)\rightarrow(0+-14\text{i})$$

5. Case of M

$$\begin{pmatrix} 2 & 4i \\ 4i & 2 \end{pmatrix}$$

$$(2+4\text{i})\times(4\text{i}+2)\rightarrow(4+8\text{i})$$

7 Conclusion

Preface

This book documents my practice of analysis over 25 years after years of training as a psychoanalytic psychotherapist and practicing in public and private settings. In contrast to my first book (2008), which failed to differentiate between hysteria and the borderline disorder, or between psychotherapy and analysis, this book only focuses on analytic cases. In addition, my last book (2021) presented more female cases of hysteria, whereas this book presents three male cases of obsessional neurosis and two cases of hysteria, one female case and one male case of hysteria, in the Lacanian sense.

I arrive at a way of quantifying psychoanalysis in mathematical and arithmetical terms that can be measured. I consider numbers that are symbolic elements appearing in dreams, fantasies, and narratives, as well as objective numbers observed in events.

I arrive at an exact number/integer for (as distinct from a quantity; see the following discussion) to 'arithmetize' symptoms and capacities. I distinguish between numbers, quantity, and images both sacred and (profane).

1. The analysand's symptoms
2. The analysand's positive capacities
3. A number that measures and predicts the capacity to recover and traverse the fantasy
4. A number that measures and predicts the capacity for high realization and functioning.

Because this is not primarily a theoretical book, it includes the psychoanalytic literature that I have often cited in other works, insofar as I use previously established analytic concepts. I also include literature on analytic processes and outcomes. However, a clinical or practice book on method is now reformulated in this book, as a mathematical discourse describable on the complex plane that measures the outcomes of psychoanalysis as a therapeutic practice.

DOI: 10.4324/9781003607038-8

This book presents a new approach that will be helpful to clinicians, analysts, supervisors, and administrators. It could be a federal model for mental health with stable long-term funding. This approach represents an effective clinical model for quality assurance and evaluating yearly outcomes, for example. I spent many years evaluating psychotherapy outcomes in a psychiatric clinic, not only to measure decreases in symptoms as a result of treatment but to also distinguish results that come from treatment and those that come from normal development and psychical resilience.

Epistemologically, psychoanalytic APA bureaucracies have regressed to statistical empiricism and reduced psychoanalysis to the large samples and statistical simplification that Freud rejected. Candidates in APA are asked about their treatment objectives with analysands. Psychanalysis was waiting for a method to be invented to measure analytic effectiveness with a mathematical method consistent with psychoanalysis.

If you wait very long for a subject to change in analysis, they may change not because of analysis but because of the passing of time. Conversely, a subject is less likely to change in a short time, so if they change, it must be because of analysis and/or another accidental factor, related to reopening critical periods in the brain. This points to the importance of transference cures at the beginning of analysis that motivate the analysand to stay in analysis and lose the money required for long-term refinance of painful personal debt.

Introduction and Methodology

This is a study of the process and outcome of singular analyses that does not rely on the methods and questionnaires of psychotherapy, or medical research.

Instead, I use abstract mathematics to make calculations that will not be based on large cardinal numbers emerging from large samples. Basic research uses probability research, for example, how many men or women suffer from depression and what type of depression. Instead, we list the symptoms as done in medical research. I want to prove the hypothesis that symptoms are cleared with the appearance of signifiers in analysis and their corresponding forms of pain and pleasure: jouissance. These signifiers, that often are names, are part of the unconscious signifying chain of a subject.

Applying the research done for a previous book (*The Jouissance of Uncountable Numbers*, 2015), I consider research on the Cartesian plane, even if used for quantum research, only appropriate for measuring symptoms, not for predicting the capacity for sublimation and positive outcomes. I argue that the latter requires the complex plane to be measured. Most people are familiar with the Cartesian plane in science but unfamiliar with the complex plane. The two planes share the x-axis and only differ by the i-axis. The i-axis is made of imaginary numbers that do not exist.

The following formula is our mathematical representation of symbolic castration, the central mathematical equation that organizes the theory.

Phi − phi = 1. The negation of the imaginary phallus: Phi − *phi*\ ; 1.618 − 0.618 = 1. I dare say that this is the equivalent of Einstein's most important equation although he was not a mathematician. This is our most important equation to characterize our use of mathematics to represent psychoanalysis. This formula is equivalent to the inhibitory function of the frontal cortex.

For each case, I arrived at a number based on both symbolic and arithmetical factors. A symbol comes out in a narrative, fantasy, or dream, and/or the number appears in symptoms and events. The imaginary that is empty, or does not exist in reality, is a measure of humanity in the good sense. The good or wholeness, or existential wholeheartedness, is the presence of emptiness, that in the mathematics of the complex plane is reached through nontrivial zeros in the imaginary axis, which I make equivalent to the Buddhist emptiness as a whole. Trivial zeros are absences and deficits as shown in symptoms and appear on the Cartesian *x*-axis. I argue that jouissance requires quantum fluctuations in the void, and that there are three of them. The first shows the farthest fluctuation from the absolute zero point, as a state of constant excitation. The second has a closer fluctuation from the void, fluctuating between excitation and release. The Third is closest to the zero of emptiness. My conceptualization relies both on mathematics and Mahayana Buddhism.

Because there are hidden (read substitutions) connections between numeric patterns/structures, not only new words or new numbers, produced by the function, but also in the phenomenological descriptions and elements, or shapes, found in biological forms and their variations, in planetary orbits and processes, and so on.

Instead of words, now we have worlds (astronomical, subatomic, biological molecular, cellular, viral, genetic). There are indeed numbers and logical connections embedded in biological forms. Since for Freud, the id was a biological substratum, perhaps he was wrong when in 1933 he said that "[t]he logical laws of thought do not apply in the Id and this is true above all of the law of contradiction" (the New Introductory Lectures, *SE*, 22, p. 73).

Contrast this with what Leibniz (1898; an earlier polymath) said in the *Theodicy*. To advance further, I want to return to the scientific work of Leibniz, a thinker who was overshadowed by Newton beating him to the publication of the calculus. Leibniz's work still undergirds the study of gravity because physics uses his notation for Newton's theory of gravity. Leibniz anticipated the dialectical logic of Hegel, but without grounding it in the pre-Socratics like Hegel and Heidegger did. Although Newton won the competition over the calculus with Leibniz, dialectical logic was a scientific discovery for Leibniz, not a historically based speculation as in Hegel.

Many judge philosophical theories in terms of idealism and realism. However, for a while now, I have argued that these categories do not apply today. Ideas are based on reality, and the Real is not reality, although all ideas come from the Real. Reality is based on images and language, and the Real is beyond both. Wrap your head around that knot.

> Our reasonings are grounded upon two great principles, that of contradiction, in virtue of which we judge false that which involves a contradiction, and true that which is opposed or contradictory to the false: (*Theodicy*, 44, 169). And that of sufficient reason, in virtue of which we hold that there can be no fact real or existing, no statement true, unless there be a sufficient reason, why it should be so and not otherwise, although these reasons usually cannot be known by us.
>
> (*Theodicy*. 44, 196)

> There are also two kinds of truths, (something Nagarjuna invented the I AD.) those of reasoning and those of fact. Truths of reasoning are necessary, and their opposite is impossible: truths of fact are contingent, and their opposite is possible. When a truth is necessary, its reason can be found by analysis, resolving it into more simple ideas and truths, until we come to those which are primary (nice description of free association).
>
> (*Theodicy*, 170, 174, 189, 280–282, 367)

It is thus that in speculative mathematics, Theorems are reduced by analysis to Axioms that are simple concepts, of which no definition can be given (i.e., emptiness); there are also first principles, which cannot be proved and indeed have no need of proof; and these are identical propositions that arise together with their opposites (*Theodicy*. 36, 37, 44, 45, 49, 52,121–122, 337, 340–344).

The truth value of Freud's statement regarding the id belongs to the logical level of impulse as experienced by a subject in society. A subject may follow the directives of the laws of desire (I want what I do not have and do not want what I have) or the law of the biological organism (hunger, for example), but the equations for these latter two conflict with the equation of what constitutes logical action in society (to use a trivial yet relevant example: to pee [p] or not pee [−p] in public).

There are numbers and logic at work in irrationality and irrational numbers despite the fact that what those numbers may represent in action may contradict what society considers logical according to other perhaps equally mathematical criteria. The irrational is not irrational but rather refers to a different form of rationality that denies the first and vice versa.

It is not the case that there is a logical system facing or interacting with another non-logical emotional system (this is only true at a phenomenological, descriptive, or existential human level). Rather, it is a matter of different logical types or levels, different levels of negation, and contradiction and non-contradiction. It is not a question of negation and no-negation or a denial of negation; it is a matter of different forms of negation: unary and binary. I believe that the concept of unary negation is one of my contributions to the field, although it is the reissuing of an ancient concept.

In unary negation, the negated remains unmarked, thus giving the impression that 'nothing' has been negated. An act or a representation has been negated, and the void or absence left in its wake, can also be negated, or replaced with a new representation. What was negated is unconscious and the unconscious appears as a void or a false hole, which itself can be negated. In a unary negation, what is negated is repressed or void, while in a binary negation, the negated is intellectually and consciously accepted.

Things, for example, can be perceived as numbers or sound waves, as music or noise, as pleasing or harsh. A harsh sound may produce a so-called irrational response such as fight or flight, attack or defend, and this may contradict a harmonious or pleasant response to sound, but in either case, a sound wave will be involved that under certain numeric conditions may produce contradictory (chaotic) or non-contradictory results (agreement or harmony).

I have shown how a function, or the Sense function can function in language and numbers. In language a function can work as sense or meaning, the latter includes censorship as a code (i.e., erase particular words/values from speech or writing) and can also be used to construct sentences and propositions. Sense or function can also be mathematical or arithmetical and refers to functions within numbers (i.e., multiplication of a number by itself). How Godel works up a code within numbers for numbers, as a form of self-consciousness.

Thus, the question can be raised whether there can be hidden connections not only between particular variables, but also between the various codes at work in nature. The objects or inputs/outputs for the function may vary, although the function always transforms one into the other for various purposes associated with the various functions.

If prime numbers are the building stones of reality, then 2, the binary that postmodern thinkers hate, is the building block of reality. The first number is 1, but it is empty in its own being and therefore equals 0 as the first script and cipher. This is a Fregean counterintuitive foundation or axiom in mathematics, like imaginary numbers are. The foundations of the Cartesian and complex planes are 2 and i, respectively.

The mathematically modeled Symbolic order, consists of the triad of Sense, or mental function, the arguments or the input/output of words/numbers and senses, and the sense objects that are apprehended by the structure as output. This is the 'what' of the structure and how the structure appears in the imaginary totality of visual perception.

Natural numbers appear to be ordered by logical or rational succession but in fact may be ordered by a ratio of irrational numbers such as the golden number or pi that continue to infinity. Mathematical structure does not exist in how numbers appear. You have to actually measure the shapes of nature and carry out arithmetical operations for the underlying so-called irrational ratio to appear.

In psychoanalysis, we do not perform arithmetical operations to reveal the irrational within the structure but rather use the rules of substitution and metaphor to arrive at the 'what' of the underlying structure that appears not to exist within the phenomenal, or manifest figures of speech and discourse. In addition, the structure can also be said to not exist in that the structure is not the same as its instantiation in the phenomenal world and is not the same as the impossible and unnamable, which are actually what we are seeking for in the search for truth and knowledge.

Of course, it all depends on how we measure effectiveness. This book offers an alternative scientific method to measure effectiveness in psychoanalysis. Finally, psychoanalysis has been repeatedly researched, yet its critics still claim that it is ineffective. Internally, its frequency has also been researched, and the study found no difference between two or three sessions per week and four or five five sessions a week (Toronto, accessed 2023). The Lacanian school in America made psychoanalysis more effective and financially affordable by accepting two to three sessions a week rather than the five to six a week practiced by IPA.

In analytic institutes, there are many who consider psychoanalytic psychotherapy more effective than psychoanalysis. Meta-studies also confirm the results obtained in other studies. However, post-analytical results continue to produce results way after the analysis has ended, thanks to Lacan's sinthome (I would add). I have written about this elsewhere (2021).

The Egyptian and Chinese Unconscious

For many years, scholars, and interested people, have been involved in an ideological controversy. Is Eastern culture collectively oriented, while the West is individualistic? Does Western psychology only apply to Europeans, or does the East have a unique manifestation of the Unconscious, or unique complexes, as some have argued? This book argues that both are true.

Freud saw psychoanalysis and dream analysis as an archeology of the mind. Therefore, in all languages, we find vestiges of other languages; in cultures, we find vestiges of other cultures; and in people and animals, we find vestiges of other beings. It is no surprise to discover that we find vestiges of Egyptian symbols in Chinese analysands, the two oldest cultures in the world, and of the history of the symbolic order, as I have called it. In all cultures, there are rudiments of mathematics and prime numbers, as seen in the examples of the Ishango bone in Africa.

The structure of language, and the structure of history is much larger than the structure of cultures and nations. Larger structures determine how different myths manifest in different cultures, more than how humans build structure in history. This is true if only because atomic and subatomic matter and particles, all the way up in steps to molecules and then to organisms, demonstrate the same structure.

This book demonstrates the effectiveness of Lacanian psychoanalysis. Issues of confidentiality are uppermost in analysis, although Freud thought that scientific discoveries are more important than issues of confidentiality. However, the practice of analysis across cultures opens fresh new challenges. The question of names is fundamental for Lacanian analysis, and they have to be analyzed despite issues of confidentiality.

Treatment of the Obsessional and Hysterical Structures

Of the six cases first discussed, three are obsessional and three hysterical. We remind the reader that for Lacan these two diagnostic structures are defined by an existential question: 'Am I a man or a woman?' 'Are you a man or a woman?' The same logic applies to the question, "Am I dead or alive?" Both structures always have symptoms and traits of the Other structure. This definition of *hysteria* differs from the *DSM*'s and Freud's. The latter define diagnoses by symptoms not questions. This is the outcome of Lacan's interest in phenomenology and the existential tradition (Sartre [atheistic] and Heidegger [nontheistic]).

Obsessional structures cannot be treated directly (pure hate) and must be 'hysterized' in the transference. The three obsessionals were successfully hysterized in the transference, while the hysteric becomes more reflective, organized, and sober. The successful 'hysterization' of the transference leads to successful treatments. The failed cases do not have to be hidden to present a successful form of treatment for mental disorders. At any point in the method, the choices are clear that lead to failed treatments. You have to be able to explain why you fail and why you succeed. An explanation that is not an uninformed opinion is episteme, Sophia, and Nous.

The borderline condition also needs to be 'neuroticized' first before analytic treatment of a neurotic can begin. The borderline becomes a neurotic rather than a psychotic or pervert and is prevented and compelled from acting out. This would require a prior treatment of psychoanalytic psychotherapy where the focus is on the first phase of the Oedipus complex and the relation to the mother's jouissance and the refusal of the paternal function.

For this chapter, I use the complex plane to trace the path of the subject through analysis. The complex plane can answer the question, 'How did the therapeutic effect take effect upon the subject?' The question of the symptom answers the question, 'What changed in analysis?' I measure symptoms in real numbers, and the capacity for sublimation is measured in imaginary numbers. Imaginary numbers allow us to see the deeper dimensions of reality such as the Buddha nature rather than simply nature.

In the past, psychoanalysis was rejected for being unscientific and for misusing the physics of the time. The rest of psychology relied on the experimental method, but more recently, psychology has relied on questionnaires and interviews. Each answer is scored from 1 to 5; the higher the number the closer it is to 1 as the truth, and most studies in medicine reach a margin of 0.025 of truth. The results are represented on the Cartesian plane. However, I argue that for psychoanalysis its efficacy is better represented by the complex plane with i numbers.

For each case I arrive (based on counting) at a metaphor, a number, and a formula to describe the subject.

For the first case, for example, his anxiety, depression, and paranoia changed. What were the signifiers that emerged in his analysis that led to the resolution of his symptoms? I argue that in some cases symptoms change and decrease as a consequence of the treatment, not only due to the passing of time. Ordinarily symptoms are measured in the clinic with simple scales. The capacity for sublimation also plays a factor in the recovery from the symptoms. 'Arithmetized', the two give us a number for the subject. Imaginary numbers have to be reduced to and revealed through the Cartesian x- and y-axes.

Table 7.1 organizes the case materials into seven categories, and I give examples while protecting confidentiality. The clinical materials are organized by themes and signifiers rather than biographical data (which also include numbers). Signifiers are singular markers of the subject's experience, rather than researcher's constructs, presented to the subject in the form of questions. I offer a rationale for the subject, or the analyst, to disclose the structure (disclose) as an aspect of the sinthome:

1. Symptoms
2. Signifiers
3. Numbers
4. Desire
5. Desire of the Other
6. Sinthome
7. Nomination

Symptoms represent both signifiers and numbers, desire is interlocked with the desire of the Other, and the sinthome is established as a process of nomination. In this sense, the table of categories constitutes a signifying chain, a causal chain, organized around a hole. The table of categories is a signifying chain of dependent origination.

For the case of S, the logical structure of the fantasy follows different content but the same process, so I keep the format the same. The same will be the case for Mario's case as well.

Table 7.1 The Chinese Unconscious

Symptoms were addressed through psychotherapy	*Diagnoses Hysterical neurosis with obsessional s.*	*Numbers*	*Signifiers are rank-ordered text*	*Desire is either 1, or signficant, or 0, or repressed*	*Desire of the Other is 1, or determining, or 0, or insignificant*	*Sinthome In i axis. Capacity for sublimation Level l of emptiness Scale 0–10i His score: 2i*	*Nomination New name of the subject or the name is resignified in analysis*
			1. Virginia				Grandpa Hao yu
1. Narcissism			2. Gigolo				Grandpa Mu
2. Irritable			3. Hole				
3. Depressed			3. Imaginary phallus/wand				
4. Hypomanic			4. Mathemes for his symptoms				
5. Insomniac			5. Circumcision				
			6. Ectonian phallus/ pregnancy				
5 × 2i Measure of pathology and capacity for sublimation			7. Government Official				

Signifiers are different from symptoms, because they form part of the unconscious signifying chain associated with the name and nomination. Symptoms are described in a simple social narrative with gaps and omissions that point to the background signifying structure.

I arrive at a metaphor and a number for each subject.

The subject's metaphor is Grandpa Wu. Wu is not only no or lack, but also the function of a unary negation. Wu in Chan means both no and yes.

The complex number of the subject is 2 × 2i.

The symptoms have lessened, although the subject began analysis with a medium capacity for sublimation. The score number is 2 in real numbers and 1 in imaginary numbers. His complex number during treatment is 2 + 2i.

For purposes of clarity, I write and view his complex number in a binary matrix. Matrix mathematics is a branch of mathematics used by Dirac to reconcile relativity theory with quantum physics. The numbers here represent the analysand (a possible card in a deck of cards), not subatomic particles and the exchangeability of electricity and magnetism. Here I am speaking of the exchangeability of suffering and drives for sublime ideals, and the assigning of a specific number to a subject. A number 2 is assigned to pathology on the reality axis and a number −2i to 'desublimation' on the imaginary axis. Marcuse's desublimation is a measure in the negative quadrant of imaginary numbers.

Using the Complex Plane to Measure Analytic Outcomes for the Singular Subject

Treatment of the obsessional and hysterical structures.

Of the six cases discussed, three are obsessional and three hysterical. We remind the reader that for Lacan these two diagnostic structures are defined by the questions, 'Am I a man or a woman?' 'Are you a man or a woman?' The same logic applies to the question, 'Am I dead or alive?' Both structures always have symptoms and traits of the Other structure. This definition of hysteria differs from the *DSM*'s and Freud's. The latter define diagnoses by symptoms, not questions.

Obsessional structures cannot be treated directly (pure hate) and must be 'hysterized' in the transference. The three obsessionals were successfully hysterized in the transference, while the hysteric becomes more reflective, organized, and sober. The successful hysterizing of the transference leads to successful treatments. The failed cases do not have to be hidden to present a successful form of treatment for mental disorders. At any point in the method, the choices that lead to failed treatments are clear. You have to be able to explain why you fail and why you succeed. An explanation that is not an uninformed opinion is episteme, Sophia, and Nous.

Now the difficulty with hysterizing one of the obsessional structures in the sample of cases is that he had a particular conflict or fear of being feminized.

So, being seductive with him and being a male analyst, he could interpret the 'histerization' as a homosexual seduction. What protected this particular analysand from that fear was a symbolic identification with psychoanalysis and Freud that protected him from this fear.

In this final chapter, I use the complex plane to trace the path of the subject through analysis. The complex plane can answer the question, 'How did the therapeutic effect take effect upon the subject?' The question of the symptom answers the question, 'What changed in analysis?' I measure symptoms in real numbers and the capacity for sublimation in imaginary numbers.

For each case, I arrive at a metaphor, a number, and a formula to describe the subject.

In the first case, for example, his anxiety, depression, and paranoia changed. What were the signifiers that emerged in his analysis that led to the resolution of his symptoms? I argue that in some cases symptoms change and decrease as a consequence of the treatment, not only due to the passing of time. Ordinarily symptoms are measured in the clinic with simple scales. The capacity for sublimation also plays a factor in the recovery from the symptoms. 'Arithmetized', the two give us a number for the subject.

A table organizes the case material into seven categories. I give examples while protecting confidentiality. The clinical material is organized by themes and signifiers rather than biographical data. Signifiers are singular markers of the experience of the subject, rather than constructs of the researcher, presented to the subject in the form of questions. I offer a rationale for the subject, or the analyst, to disclose the structure (disclose – not advertise) as an aspect of the sinthome.

1. Symptoms
2. Signifiers
3. Numbers
4. Desire
5. Desire of the Other
6. Sinthome
7. Nomination

Symptoms represent both signifiers and numbers, desire is interlocked with the desire of the Other, and the sinthome is established as a process of nomination. In this sense, the table of categories constitutes a signifying chain, a causal chain, organized around a hole. The table of categories is a signifying chain of dependent origination.

For the case of S, the logical structure of the fantasy uses different content but the same process, so I keep the format the same. The same is used for Martin's case as well.

Signifiers are different from symptoms because they form part of the unconscious signifying chain associated with the name and nomination.

I try to arrive at a metaphor and a number for each subject.

Table 7.2 Chinese Case

Symptoms were addressed through psychotherapy	*Diagnoses Hysterical neurosis with obsessional sx.*	*Numbers*	*Signifiers are rank-ordered in the text*	*Desire Is either 1, or significant, or 0, or repressed*	*Desire of the Other is 1, or determining, or 0, or insignificant*	*Sinthome on i-axis. Capacity for sublimation Level of emptiness 0 to 10i His score: 2i*	*Nomination New name of the subject or the name is resignified in analysis*
			8. Virginia				Grandpa Haoyu
1. Narcissism			9. Gigolo				Grandpa Mu
2. Irritable			3. Hole				
3. Depressed			10. Imaginary phallus/wand				
4. Hypomanic			11. Mathemes for his symptoms				
5. Insomniac			12. Circumscision				
			13. Ectonian				
5 × 2i			14. Government official				
Measure of pathology and capacity for sublimation							

The subject's metaphor is Grandpa Wu. Wu is not only no or lack but also the function of a unary negation.

The number of the subject in the complex plane is 2 × 2i.

The symptoms have gone down, although the subject began analysis with a low capacity for sublimation. The score number is 2 in real numbers and 1i in imaginary numbers. His complex number during treatment is 2 + 2i.

For purposes of clarity, I write and view his complex number in a binary matrix. Matrix mathematics is a branch of mathematics used by Dirac to reconcile relativity theory with quantum physics. The numbers here represent the analysand, not subatomic particles and the exchangeability of electricity and magnetism. Here I am speaking of the exchangeability of suffering, drives for sublime ideals, and assigning a specific number to a subject. A number 2 is assigned to pathology on the reality Cartesian axis and a number −2i to 'desublimation' in the imaginary axis.

Repressive desublimation, a term first coined by Frankfurt school philosopher and sociologist Herbert Marcuse in his 1964 work *One-Dimensional Man*, refers to the way in which, in advanced industrial society (capitalism), the progress of technological rationality is liquidating the oppositional and transcending elements in the 'higher culture'. The higher culture is getting desublimated. Finally, the discourse of the capitalist is the discourse where the subject completes themselves through consumption, and the science and knowledge about the objects of consumption also lead to increased consumption. Lacan calls the *objet a* a 'lathouse' to refer to the use of computers and internet-based information and AI to impact consumption and economic exchange. The information about the *objet a* is Imaginary, but it facilitates economic exchange.

Continuing with his formula,

$$\begin{pmatrix} 2 & -2i \\ 2i & 2 \end{pmatrix}$$

$$(2+-2\mathrm{i})\times(2\mathrm{i}+2)\rightarrow(4+4\mathrm{i})\,.$$

In this case, the subject's complex number is 4 + 4i emerging from the core of their being, or, in other words, the core of the axis. Complex numbers have a wave function from 2, −2 to 4, –4 and so on).

Maxwell used matrix mathematics to describe the exchangeability of electricity and magnetism. To obtain a single matrix equation instead of a pair, new functions were constructed using the components of the Riemann–Silberstein vector. For Riemann (1854), geometry is about calculating the length of every curve. It is unclear to me how the study of spheres and circles was a mystical concern of Pythagoras in antiquity that continued into the Middle Ages, but somehow modern geometry is different from that? It turns out that the new geometry is very much like the old geometry calls out the outlines and limits of coastlines and the shapes of leaves 'as if' out of nowhere.

I am sure that this statement reflects my ignorance of how the two geometries understand triangles and angles differently. Nevertheless, I use matrix mathematics to describe the exchangeability of the signifier, for images, and for images for jouissance. $(S \rightarrow I \rightarrow R = X \rightarrow Y \rightarrow Z)$. RSI (Real, Symbolic, Imaginary) is the function of XYZ.

Jouissance has acceleration in the displacement from signifier to signifier, while jouissance can also be condensed in a metaphor. Conversely, magnetism can be condensed in a chain of metaphors or can represent the condensed Real beyond or outside representation. Is the radiation associated with magnetism damaging, or medically therapeutic? Using radiation in war is damaging, while in a small dose, it is positive. Positive and negative charges repel each other, and this is how magnetism controls for gravity.

Is there anything spiritual about magnetism? Is magnetism the mind equivalent of the concentration of samadhi or even the Sabbath (*Samedi*). It all depends on the color (quantity) of energy concentration (blue is cool and low entropy, heat is red, and the spectrum in between these two colors is purple). Nirvana is blue and cool, and fire and light are pure energy, yellow and red, respectively. Purple is the color of nobility of spirit. Blue is calm, and red is passion and compassion. Magnetism is what stops you when you move or fall (think of a free climber depending on the magnetism between their fingers and the fractal shape of the mountainside). Stopping is the same as calmness of mind and non-movement. You stay calm because you do not move, and because your body-mind does not move, you can travel fast. The universe is accelerating, and at the same time, it does not move and stays in the same place.

Cxyz is the complex subjugation of SIR (Symbolic, Imaginary, Real) into the quantifying triplet, and $M = [M_x, M_y, M_z]$ is a vector whose component permuting elements are abstract as 4×4 matrices have shown. We have RSI, ISR, SIR, SIR, and the sinthome.

From the component M-matrices, we get

$$\Omega \quad \begin{matrix} [0 & -I_2] \\ [I_2 & o] \end{matrix}$$

$$\beta \quad \begin{matrix} [2i & 0] \\ [0 & 2i]] \end{matrix} .$$

Alpha (the center of the *x*- and i-planes) and Omega represent the wave function and the infinite straight line emerging from the center of the plane, which is the objective equivalent of the subjective center of a subject.

The subject of the complex plane is both a subject and an object in a dialectical moment as Freud, Jung, and their followers believed.

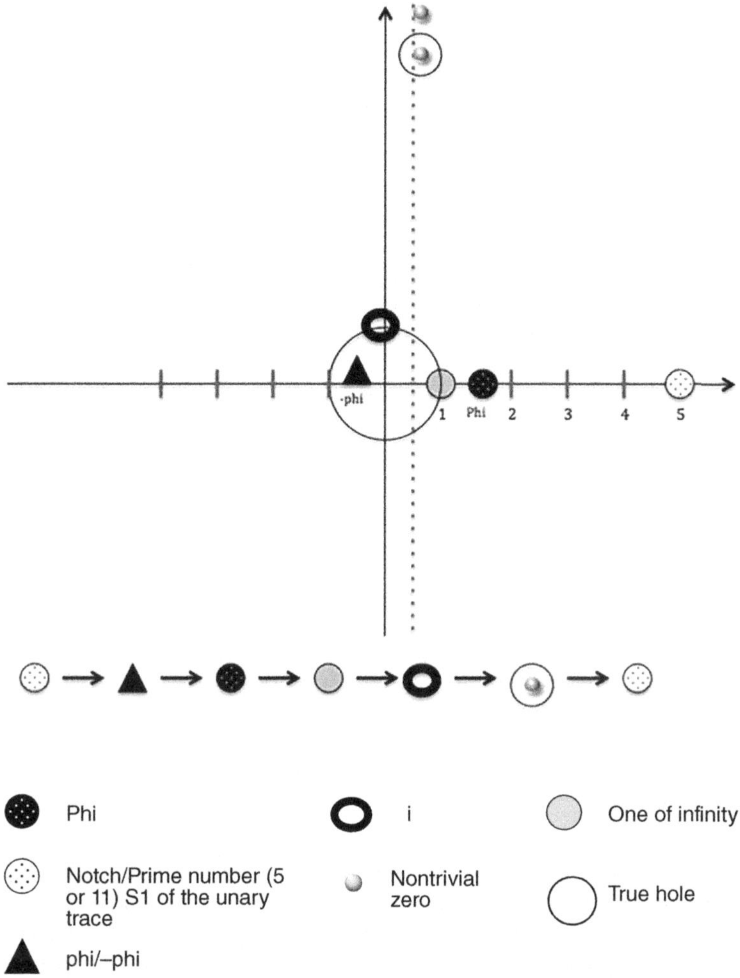

Figure 7.1 The component M-matrices

We see in the Figure 7.1 that the complex plane looks like the Cartesian plane, except that the numbers differ and signify the different circles which represent symbolic positions.

A tensor in physics, for example, has four component elements, revealing a formal structure and order at the microparticle level. Ordinarily, the macro level represents order, and the micro level represents disorder. Here, the micro is orderly while the macro is disorderly. What are the implications of this? Well, usually the small, or the leader, is controlled by the large, although the subjective experience of the leader and group members may be the reverse. In this case, however, the large, or the group is also controlled by the leader or the small. For psychoanalysis, the small is the *objet a*, expressed as a tensor. Why is the *objet a* organizing rather than disorganizing? Rotation around a centripetal hole, for example, structures the elliptical orbits of the planets. A tensor is effective in counting the sexual tension inside a subject in relation to the object causing desire.

The micro is like the order of RSI installed at a microparticle level with 0 and 1 as imaginary numbers, in addition to the 0 and 1 of real numbers. The fourth element I name the third jouissance, a convenient positive feeling state or sense of well-being that is immeasurable and nonnumerical (1 = R).

There is a positive and a negative 1. The Real is the 1 that is 0 or a 0 that is a 1. The Imaginary is the 1 that is 1. Then there also two zeros: the zero of absence and the zero of presence. Zero is the signifier of desire and lack (S); 0′ is suffering or pain, as a negative absence (Imaginary −phi or −0.68 . . .), and another 0 as a sense of well-being derives from emptiness.

From 0 as a signifier of desire or lack, and the imaginary phallus as virtual source of suffering, for Lacan the ψ phallus also appears as a golden number in the form of 0.68. In the matrix, the phi could also be represented as a temperature or heat tensor and how a vernacular use of language links heat to sexuality. A heat tensor for a subject would pair the heat of the drive (nature) with the heat of ideals (the burning bush) in the biblical burning bush.

$$(4 \times 4i)$$

$$(-4 \quad 4)$$

These four elements also correspond to the four levels of the signifiers: the trace/trait lower unit of the signifier, the letter, the word, and the sentence. The four positive and negative elements interact within the matrix, generating the formal structure of the thinking that determines the subject's experience, as well as the outside that organizes the order and cohesion of the structure. Here, the theory is formally modeled after mathematics, but the arithmetization still has to be proven by being replicated and validated by real mathematicians. My use of abstract mathematics, although accurate, is intuitive or philosophical but is not a mystical use of numbers as in Jewish or Christian gematria and/or numerology.

The 1 in the matrices are imaginary numbers. What does it mean in this model that sublimation is described by imaginary numbers that do not exist? In addition, the 0s can be the 0 of the Cartesian plane or the 0 of the complex plane. This real 0 also differs from the nontrivial 0s that appear in the critical

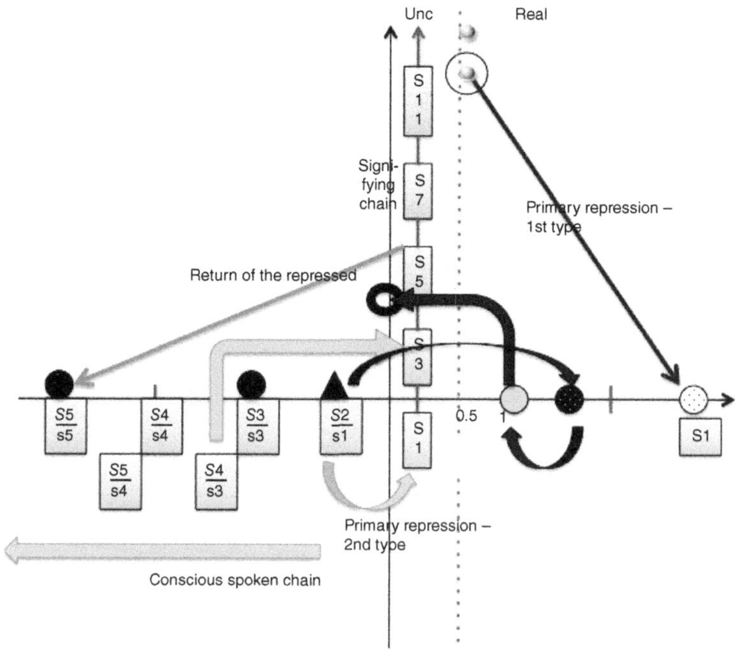

Figure 7.2 A list of symptoms, diagnosis, numbers, desire of the Other, sinthome, and nomination

line (0.5) along the i-axis of imaginary numbers. Trivial 0s appear on the real x-axis (Fig. 7.2).

Sublimation is a different negativity (−1) than the negativity of negative x numbers in the Cartesian plane. Sublimation is a positive negativity that differs from repression or is a different type of repression. Sublimation is based on a primary form of repression in the Real unconscious that is not oppressive. We do not know 'it' or repress/forget it because it is a Real outside representation.

In the case of this Chinese subject, the i of imaginary numbers is low, or a small number, as shown in this graph. We see that in the negative x-axis the numbers come in pairs of signifier/signified. On the positive side of the x-axis, prime numbers appear. In our cases, only two cases generated the prime numbers 5 and 7. Prime numbers are what build structure, so these case examples happen to be of leaders in a field of knowledge.

The subject's metaphor: the One who bears.

His complex number after treatment is 1 × 2i.

Table 7.3 Case of S

Symptoms	*Diagnoses*	*Ranked signifiers*	*Numbers Total 6*	*Desire 1 or 0*	*Desire of Other 1 or 0*	*Sinthome*	*Nomination*
1. Depression	Obsessional neurosis with hysterical symptoms	1. My son the doctor 2. My son the criminal		1. To be a man. Fuck 1 or 2	1. That he be a man	He is a sinner/saint who 'fucks' paternal grandmother (2 1i) (1i 2)	the One who bears
2. Anxiety		S. the snake, the player		Kill the father steal the breast			
3. Fear 4. Being minority 5. Paranoia							

Formula for the subject: The complex number read as a binary matrix and represented in a graph:

$$\begin{pmatrix} 1 & -2i \\ 2i & 1 \end{pmatrix}$$

$$(1+-2i)\times(2i+1)\rightarrow(2+4\mathrm{i})$$

Complex numbers convert the false hole into the true hole, the emptiness of absence into the emptiness of presence, and calculate the level of emptiness (depression), and the level of sublimation. Take for example, a subject with symptoms yet a high spiritual or aesthetic capacity for sublimation in art or mathematics (Table 7.3).

Metaphor of the subject: the Martyr.

Number for the subject is 3 × 2i.

Formula for the subject:

$$\begin{pmatrix} 1^{\cdot} & -2i \\ -2i & 1 \end{pmatrix}$$

$$(1+-2\mathrm{i})\times(-2\mathrm{i}+1)\rightarrow(2+-4\mathrm{i})$$

Metaphor of the subject: the spirit of truth.

The number for the subject is 0 × 7i.

The formula for the subject:

$$\begin{pmatrix} 0 & -7i \\ -7i & 0 \end{pmatrix}$$

$$(0+-7)\times(-7+0)\rightarrow(0+-14\mathrm{i})$$

The metaphor of the subject: The name as a light in a man: The ‘holy’ dark light in your eyes

The number of the subject is 2 × 5i.

The formula for the subject:

$$\begin{pmatrix} 2 & 4i \\ 4i & 2 \end{pmatrix}$$

$$(2+4\mathrm{i})\times(4\mathrm{i}+2)\rightarrow(4+8\mathrm{i})$$

Table 7.4 Case of Martin

Symptoms	*Diagnoses*	*Ranked signifiers*	*Numbers*	*desire*	*Desire of Other*	*Sinthome*	*Nomination*
1. Anxiety	Hysterical neurosis with obsessional symptoms	My son the bohemian		1. To be a woman	He has to account for himself. That he be special	He is a sinner/ saint pervert who wants to kill his father	The Martyr
2. Malevolent depersonalization							
3. Addiction							
Complex score 3 × 2i		After treatment 1 × 2i Psychoanalysis is the ideal but is no longer idealized	1 Not a prime number although it is the origin of numbers.			2i	

Table 7.5 Literary Benevolence

Symptoms	*Diagnoses*	*Ranked signifiers*	*Numbers*	*desire*	*Desire of Other*	*Sinthome*	*Nomination*
1. Anxiety	Obsessional structure with hysterical symptoms.	1. Peachy	3 and 7 = 10	1. little devil	That he be special boy 1	He is a sinner with women	1. Son of the Buddha: Rahul 2. Moncayo. The name of a mountain in Spain.
2. Am I dead?		2. My son the handsome scholar		2. To be a Buddha	He writes like the greats	Mystic third jouissance and jouissance of meaning	2. The empty mountain spirit of truth
		3. You shall amount to ‘nothing’ like my brother Augustus					
Before treatment 2 × 3i	After treatment	0 × 7i 7i out of 10	7 Is a prime number				

Table 7.6 Case of M

Symptoms	*Diagnoses*	*Ranked signifiers*	*Numbers*	*Desire*	*Desire of Other*	*Sinthome*	*Nomination*
1. Anxiety	Hysterical neurosis with obsessional symptoms	My son the scholar. Traumatic mother's gaze takes son's picture	4	To be a boy 1	That he be special boy He completes both parents	He is a boy addicted to mother's breast	Yin The 'holy' dark light in your eyes
2. I am and my father is a woman						Feminine third jouissance	
2. I and father are crazy		4 × 3i =				3i	
3. Depersonalization							
4. Addiction		After treatment 2 + 4i					

The score of the treatment indicates the level of recovery and the potential for higher functioning. If the x-xis numbers remain high and the i numbers remain low, then the chances of change are also low.

The higher the i score, the higher the potential for the subject to be a successful professional, or analyst, a true teacher, or scholar. In this case, the subject is a senior analyst who has reached a 7 in a total score of 10. A total score of 10 would be unreachable perfection.

The case of "in you" more than you.

New name from the Real is resignified as 'in-you' because the name in Chinese also means 'in'. The other name means 'foreign' or 'out'.

The name is symptom, the supplement of dependence on the man (male or female) to become a strong man like the problem with hysterical dependence on names to be strong. Now with the new name of 'in-you', you have a relationship to the Name and the symbolic phallus in the form of the *objet a* as eyes as 'in-you' as a woman. The strength of the imaginary phallus that you lack, you search for in the dependence to the name or the man.

I am really impressed by your interpretation, Raul. No word can express my feelings at this moment. What I may respond is maybe 'It's just like This'. It seems that you find out that exact me in me. The other day you mentioned my family name as 'in-you'. I was impressed by your connection then because the sliding sound from 'in' to 'you' in English is very similar to the Chinese pronunciation of my name and most importantly, the sound from 'in' to 'you' also corresponds to the exact meaning of 于 in Chinese 'in something or related to something'. 'New Name from the Real' reminds me of Joyce and his mention of epiphany. Yes, this is a moment of epiphany for me. The new name from the Real is the NoF from the Real. Thank you for leading me there.

I was especially shocked by your interpretation of my symptom. You make what you said yesterday more clearly to me here. Thank you for that. Yesterday when you mentioned several names, I've already received the message. It produced a great therapeutic effect upon me. And I had a dream this early morning where my high school class teacher appeared. She shared the same name with my mom, a kind of flower. Yes, my name is always my symptom, symbolizing something problematic with the side of masculinity in me.

This is why Nan Huaijin (南怀瑾), a famous Chinese cultural scholar for I-Ching (易经) warned people not to study yin–yang philosophy. You helped me get an intimate touch with it. That is an amazing journey full of Lacan's detours and Godel's twists. But different from Nan Huaijin's worries, I believe that the destination is very clear: it will lead to more discoveries, beautiful and inspiring in every sense.

Phoneme is based on sound. 'In you' is like a sound that is like drawing a circle in the air that represents the wave of sound as a traceless trace that erases the trace of the symptom through a homophone. The wave of sound then is interpreted as 'just this' and 'just this' is represented as a form of the third jouissance. Russell said the first names like John or Mary means 'just this' as a singularity of jouissance rather than a particular person.

With the gaze and the eye, we also have a wave of light, so the light in you, that you get back from using me as objet a of the gaze. The eyes in you, the pearl in you that you saw in the form of the Other's gaze, comes back to you as inner light, or the inward light.

'Thank you very much, Raul, for the further explanation. phoneme is based on sound. In you is like a sound that is like drawing a circle in the air that represents the wave of sound as a traceless trace.'

Russell said the first names like John or Mary mean 'just this', as a singularity of jouissance rather than a particular person. This part is quite mystic, Raul. But since you lead me to feel it more and more in analysis, I know what you are saying. It's a knowing upon non-knowing. It just happened. Word fails to explain it, but sound is so full at the moment. Sound is the intangible Real. It impowers the signifying chain to run only on the level of the signifiers by turning itself into phoneme and creating new signifiers and in this way the symptom as the signifed inscribed in the body, is emptied of its meaning and therefore falls off from its original signifiers.

This analysand symptoms were anxiety, jealousy and envy for which I give her −2i. Her abilities included high intelligence and spirituality, so I gave her 5i. Through analysis, her score went up from −2 to 3i. Her abilities helped her wake up in analysis to 6i.

Case of T

T is a very attractive 40-year-old highly educated professional woman self-described as a feminist.

The request for analysis was expressed in terms of her desire to understand what happened with the failure of her first marriage, seeking relief from the guilt she felt over this and the problem represented by a very disturbed daughter of her current partner. She also reported a problem with a generalized sense of anxiety.

With her first husband, she married a man who was very successful, attractive, experienced, and very popular with women. Initially she said that the marriage failed because neither believed in fidelity, and the marriage ended when she left her husband for one of her lovers.

At the outset of analysis, she wanted to let me know that infidelity was not a problem for her, that she did not see it as a symptom and that she justified it in terms of a feminist ideology that a woman's body is not a man's property. She was speaking to the Other, the father, who could judge her, lay down the law or embody the guilt and the very much fought against sense of debt toward her first husband. As is always the case in analysis gradually in time the story changes as hidden and censored details, fantasies, memories, and signifiers emerge. The no-law of the analyst emerges as the censored law operating within the subject.

T did not believe in fidelity, because the mother had suffered for her sexual fidelity to the father. Because of being faithful, her mother did not left her father, although he was obnoxious, domineering, and right wing. But the father was lacking in intelligence and education. There was an imaginary father; there was also a symbolic lacking father, but it could not symbolize the lack in the father. Nor could she or her mother symbolize the lack in the mother because her mother was perceived as perfect and the father as unworthy. Had her father been educated, then she could symbolized his lack, her mother's, and her own. She did not believe in tying herself down to any man. She was her own best man.

With her first husband she did not feel pleasure and she either felt nothing or sex was painful. He was a Don Juan type who wanted to show his sexual prowess, and although allegedly neither of them believed in marital fidelity, when she finally left him for her current partner, he became unglued to the point of suicidality and suicide threats. She also disliked the desire that he had for her recognition of his sexual and intellectual prowess.

Another thing that emerged in the course of analysis is that with some trepidation she disclosed that she never wanted to have children. Again, like with the question of fidelity, she did not want this seen as a symptom, although again when the law was not forthcoming from me, she wondered several times that maybe she should have children. As an explanation and justification for not having children she quoted her mother who always told her that although she loved her and her brothers she would have preferred to have not had children and dedicated herself to her career. Her father has asked her for grandchildren and often when she was an adolescent wanted her to be a decent girl and not a "prostitute" and not to wear miniskirts or stay out late, although when she did it anyway, he looked the other way. Her mother felt tied down to her father, who was considered a very good provider and sexual partner but a burden nonetheless. Her father was not educated, and her mother had a PhD. Her mother is described as more intelligent than her father. In addition, he had a bad temper and very right-wing political beliefs. He is said to have adored her mother, and no complaints are given of her.

The reason T herself gives for not wanting children is due to all the service work required. However, another complaint was that she provided too much service to friends, coworkers, and others; was never being able to say no; and was always being taken advantage of. In other words, service is a kind of jouissance to her. She met her current boyfriend when they were both married, and both left their spouses. He was married to a woman 15 years older than him and has a daughter who became severely anorexic, bulimic, a cutter, and suicidal with her parents' divorce. The daughter requires constant supervision, and the father is totally at her bequest and has reassured patient that he will do all the work and that she will not have to do any. Now T is going to live with him, and so will the daughter, so T feels haunted by having to have a daughter she did not want and who requires an absolute form of service.

T's partner is loyal to her, but she has told him that she does not believe in fidelity, and he tolerates this but is not pleased. She describes their sexual relationship as very enjoyable although when they are apart, she does not miss him and instead fantasizes about another man with the return of her partner being a spoiler of the party. However, she is very dependent on being loved by the boyfriend and does not want to leave him or be left by him. At times she also expressed the desire that her partner would limit her excess. Recently, she met a younger man who did not succumb to her advances, and this was very destabilizing for her. Every now and then she comes to her sessions with microskirts, and she lifts her legs while on the couch.

Recently, with much embarrassment and reluctance to explore and associate with the material, she disclosed that during sex, they role-play her fantasies where he is with another woman or she is with another man or where she is another anonymous woman who sometimes is a prostitute. The disclosure of these fantasies was prefaced by apologies and justifications that fantasies are a normal part of the sexual relationship. In other words, fantasies sustain desire. On the other hand, the way that fantasies are symptoms that defend against castration is not something that she yet can consider.

She further disclosed with vulnerability and without apology or justification prostitution fantasies which are masturbatory in nature where she is a prostitute to a line of men who want her service, and she very much wants to satisfy all their fantasies and desires.

In a dream, T is with many naked men among them is her ex-husband. He has an erection, but the penis is facing down. She then begins to spin like Clark Kent does to turn into Super-Man and becomes a superwoman.

Associations: She is one of the men. She always likes being among groups of men and feeling like she is one of them. Cartoon of a little girl who transforms into a supergirl or heroine. The lowered erection makes it less threatening and intrusive. The inverted male sign is a symbol used by feminists. During puberty, she was embarrassed about having breasts, and she would wear special clothing to disguise them. Growing up, she wanted to be a boy and not a girl. She did not want to have breasts, did not play with dolls, and was a tomboy. She had a profound disgust and fear of menstruation.

Termination

Feelings and thoughts about it. No, will work on it with Hans in Mexico. Her analysis will not end because she will continue with herself analysis. The other is not symbolized. The other is either replaced by a substitute or by herself. She talks about herself but not to me. Or she talks to me but not about herself but about me and my shortcomings. For example, when she referred to my speaking too much or more than her previous analyst or how she liked an analyst in Mexico. This is the place of the analyst as the man who "*no sirve*" (it is useless), good for nothing, Lacanian analysis does not work or does not function, is impotent. Then there is the judge, as described earlier. With me, she respected analysis once again. Remembered that as a girl when she was deprived of something, a girl not letting her play with a doll, her attitude was, this does not affect me.

Discussion

Growing up, she wanted to be a man and not a woman. The presence of breasts was a minus, an absence, a sign of a loss in the gaze of the Other. More than as an *objet a* that covers a hole, the breast was the signifier of the minus phi, of the lack, of not having the phallus. This meaning of wounding loss was further emphasized by the disgust towards bleeding from her genitals in menstruation.

She found her first husband threatening. His erect penis was feared and wounding. Although he was quite a catch for her, she found his demand to be recognized as a master, annoying and demeaning. In Hegelian fashion, the master needs a servant to recognize them as a master; the slavery of the master and the mastery of the servant are revealed at the end of their relationship, which leaves her with remorse for having destroyed him.

T wanted to be a man or a superwoman but not the woman as the signifier of symbolic castration, of the lack in the Other. To be a professional woman, she did not need to be a man because she was encouraged to study by both parents and mother was already a successful academic. In her mind, a woman corresponded to being a wife and a mother but not at the exclusion of being a professional woman or an intellectual. This is the place where she refuses symbolic castration and sexual difference under the fear of the imaginary father/phallus experienced as an imaginary form of castration as in the example of having breasts, menstruation, and children. Having means not having.

The disavowed symbolic femininity returns in the Imaginary and the Real. In the Real of jouissance she is always having to be a servant to other women, and she fears she will end up being the hyper-servant of the grotesque and uncanny daughter she did not want. In the Imaginary she enjoys being of service and a sexual servant of many men so long as she is not limited to serving only one man. If her partner is of service to her or his daughter, this causes her to look elsewhere for the man who may have another woman instead of serving her. The service of the man is seen as an imaginary form of castration. The service of the man means both the man serving her and her serving the man.

Her desire is for the desire of the mother. This is the mother of the Imaginary and not of the Symbolic mother. The maternal gift is not absent. The mother makes herself absent as a mother in the sense that she desires things beyond the child but remains in a position of omnipotence. Such omnipotence is limited by the imaginary father but not in the sense of the idealized father but in the sense of the brutal father (yells, farts, and makes arbitrary demands at times) and of the father who desires and gives satisfaction to the mother.

The mother enjoyed sex with the father and in fact it was so good that she felt that this enjoyment enslaved her to him because otherwise she would have left him. But there is no imaginary idealized father or the ideal of a symbolic father sustained by the emptiness of the function. This is directly related to the metaphor of the father in the mother's speech. The mother appears as omnipotent and the father as a burden. T stays in the position of identification with and being the cause of the mother's desire. Her desire is not completely displaced in the direction of finding and avowing the law of the father that then could lead to an idealization of the father and then to a falling off from this idealization. Her phantasm fills the lack in the Other in that she identifies with the omnipotent mother and searches for the idealized non-lacking father which defends against the presence of femininity which could serve as a guarantor of the emptiness of the symbolic phallus function.

The mother does not take care of the father; the father wants to leave because the mother is fat.

What she thinks of herself	*What the other thinks of her*
Here she does not know what to say. Perhaps give a class that nobody has given before.	Female students say that gives the best class. This is what she is capable of doing with her body.
She constantly loses her thesis.	In Mexico, the old men of academia don't like her.
She cannot have the symbolic phallus.	

'The construction of femininity: The spectacle of my body and its potency. The gaze of mothers. In the dance everything goes and then it ends. I am the dream of my mother, her with her polio and her fat body'. Father sin and agile, and a good lover. The competition with males began at home. Weaning, and rejection, the perception of weakness, the ideal of masculinity the competition with h brothers.

In her case, she had anxiety but was not high; otherwise, she was not symptomatic. So, we gave her a −2 for anxiety, and grief as an expression of the perceived lack of femininity. Because she had a high level of education, we also gave her a 3i. Her capacity for analysis allows her to change. She met these objectives at the end of the personal analysis and went from −2i to 2i, and from 3i to 5i.

In the case of another analysand, he had a dream that provides a good example of the agalma. He was in a synagogue with altar in Jerusalem. He was the rabbi/teacher. He opens a secret box that has a cardboard with Hebrew letters. The letters have extreme power, although he does not know what they mean. In the next scene, he is holding a stone called the tiger's eye. He wants to tell me he is leaving and asks me what the letters mean. I tell him it is the name of my grandfather, Levi Yitzchak, who meditated on his own name.

He wants to smuggle the rock back into the US, he flirts with my wife and becomes afraid that Arabs may stab him.

At first the agalma appears in its entire splendor: the holy and awesome setting, the sense of spiritual delight and the mysterious, the signifiers of the symbolic father, and the precious stone or jewel. The phallic and narcissistic significance of the agalma is only secondarily revealed when the letters without a fixed signification become the letters that he attributed to the name of my grandfather, who was supposed to have used them to meditate on his own name. For Jews this would be a heretical act given that Jews only meditate on the Tetragrammaton (the four-lettered name of G-d), the meaning of which remains unknown. In addition, the reference to his grandfather meditating on his own name was linked by association to the fact that this analysand engaged in a ritual act of performing fellatio on himself. The alleged name of his grandfather stands as a signifier of the imaginary father/phallus. He then tries to steal (smuggle) the imaginary phallus and use it to flirt with his wife. The aggressive nature of the act is revealed by the projective or paranoid fear of Arabs.

Socrates professed no knowledge except that of his own not knowing. He believed that people know both less and more than what they think they do. To those who appeared to know he showed them that they actually did not know; and to those who appeared not to know, he showed them that in fact they did know: 'This object that you apparently want from me and that you think I have, is your own object. Not that you have it or are it, but "it" lives in you, as your own fantasy.' Lacan compared Socrates's response to the subjective position of the analyst or to what Lacan called the desire of the analyst.

An analysand had a vision, it was the evening of his wedding in 1985. Suddenly he spontaneously entered in a state of bliss that I knew from the earlier experience of circumcision. Then the space around him disappeared and he was in empty space and in front of me appeared a marble stairway leading up to a platform where stood an old man with a long beard dressed in a white robe and in a very equanimous state. Most strikingly behind him there was a full moon shining like the sun.

From there he went to the place where the wedding was going to take place, and upon entering, he encountered a lay rabbi who looked just like the old man on the platform.

The second vision was when he went to Israel. At the beginning of Shabbat HaGadol, he walked down to the Temple in Jerusalem. Shabbat HaGadol is a sabbath of consolation, after the 11th of Av when the second temple was destroyed. He was born on the 9th of Av or July 30. As he approached the Wailing Wall, his mind went into a state of deep bliss and radiance, and when he looked up the Wall at the top and the meeting place of the Wall and heaven, he saw the same full moon shining like the sun.

in a third vision, he was the retreat director at the Berkeley Zen Center, sitting in the front seat. In the afternoon, during an open period of meditation, the sesshin director also sat facing the wall, rather than sitting facing the community of practitioners. Against the wall appeared the full moon shining like the sun with two Hindu figures by the side engaged in a sacred dance. The G-d of enlightenment or brightness according to the Kabbalah, is both Jewish and Hindu, according to his visions. Hinduism historically came before Judaism, although it may come after Abraham as described in the Bible.

The sun is the source of light not only as an object but as a condensation of energy present in all things. The sun shining like the moon is also a metaphor of inner subjective and mental life.

He struggled a lot with conflicting relative loyalties to Zen Buddhism and Judaism, whether he needed to decide between one or the other, conflicts with his wife over this, and the issues of identity that this brought up. He felt very drawn to Judaism, because of the spirituality mentioned earlier, but felt that these Jewish experiences were influenced and made possible by Zen experience that he was not ready to give up.

A lot of other Jews did not seem to be having these experiences. At one point, after he returned from a trip to Israel, he went back to the Zen center, and before going in he asked Buddha in heaven for a very clear sign that Zen practice was for him and that he should stay with it. If he did not get this sign, he was prepared to abandon the practice. Once he took a seat in the Zendo or meditation hall, he entered a very deep samadhi (an experience that has preceded all of the visionary and deep spiritual experiences he has had) or state of calm luminous concentration and bliss, and then somehow, he found himself up in the air in the middle of the room with Mel, and their bodies, in the lotus posture, went right through one another in absolute transparency. This was an experiential realization of the teaching of interdependence. Their bodies fused and passed through each other without obstacle. It was interesting that this was an instance during which a supplicative prayer to the Jewish absolute did work, yet he received a Buddhist response to the prayer from a Jewish Zen teacher. So 'who' was listening? It was 'Juda Buddha', the Tathagata.

Low-Heeled Shoes as a Mark of Femininity

This is a woman in her late 30s, who just finished four years of analysis on online video, occasional phone sessions at times, with office sessions once at the beginning of the analysis and then another set of sessions in the middle phase of the analysis. The analysis ended online.

Half of my work at this point is online or on the phone; the other half is in the office. I work with people in different parts of the country and in different countries, mostly in English. I began working online once I became a control analyst 11 years ago. I worked as a psychologist/psychotherapist for 10 years, and then as an analyst in formation for about 7 years all in the office. I had worked as a supervisor for decades before that, and as director of training in a large psychiatric clinic.

In the office, the analysand enters the office and lies down on the couch with the analyst behind them. If the patient prefers, the analysis can begin face-to-face at first during the preliminary sessions until they decide to work together.

Online, we meet via videoconference, and at first, if there is any business, it is okay to start face-to-face in the office or online.

Once the analysand lies down, the analyst is at the computer behind the couch. Or if this is not possible, the analysand lies down with their feet resting on an Ottoman chair if not a couch and the turns off their video. Analysis can also be done over the phone.

For this case presentation, the initial presentation of symptoms was vague, and it was unclear what she wanted to keep, what she wanted to change, and if her jouissance was pleasure or suffering. Symptoms and fantasies emerged in the analysis over time, and they were embedded in her character traits.

Character traits are usually in the body: a stiff upper lip, a nervous gesture, or copying somebody else's style of speaking.

Character traits are either egosyntonic or egodystonic. *Egodystonic* means that problems are problems for others but not for the ego. The ego loves its traits that are a problem for others.

Symptoms rather than character traits are always ego-dystonic because they cause pain for the subject.

Symptoms

1. 'Anxiety is stirred up in the core of my being' with respect to a man she was seeing briefly when she began the analysis. 'I just want to be close to him, to ravish him, to make him love me'.

   I must warn you that I use the foul language the analysand used. Analysts have to use this language, not only because it contains lalangue (language of the unconscious – for example, 'motherfucker') but because we are like medical doctors who need to work with the body without standards of proper social speech getting in the way.

   'I know that fucking someone the way I fucked him isn't the way girls get boys to love them'. She rejects passive femininity.
2. She said that relationship with her father did not provide sustenance and was harmful.

   It was difficult for her to imagine herself in a long-term relationship. The first sexual difference is with the father and then in latency is transferred to other boys, and in puberty it becomes sexual.

   'The closest was thinking of buying a duplex with me living next door to the person, something that could point to something lasting, but it never played itself out'.
3. She gets angry and jealous in relationships. She thought he was interested in other women. She had an elaborate fantasy with a friend of his. He never met her; he lived in Los Angeles, and nothing was going on between them.

She feared losing him to another woman. It had something to do with going back to using drugs.

She has a history of drug use since she ran away from home at age 12 and dropped out of school. She prostituted herself a few times to obtain drugs and spent a total of 5 years in prison due to stealing and committing fraud to obtain drugs.

She became sober through Narcotics Anonymous and was already sober when she started her analysis. She finished her high school and college in prison and was in a PhD program in women's studies when she started her analysis, was dissatisfied with North American gender studies, and came looking for Lacanian psychoanalysis, which is a slowly but surely growing trend in the United States.

4. She is so malleable and has no identity

   She became what everyone around her was, and she idealized men and fetishized them. Resist white middle-class shit in the university. Idealized street credibility

   She rejects trashy and respectability. She occupies a space in the middle and does not fit in in either place. Does not know what identity she wants to affirm.

   Lacan said the woman does not exist in the Symbolic only 'ex-sists' in the Real, so she has the flexibility or the disorientation to be an Other woman or the ideal woman.

Family History

Her parents had her when they were 18 and were not married. Her mother's family did not like her father, who was bright and handsome but a recluse and antisocial, fitting a character type not uncommon in the US known as a survivalist. Poor whites are retreating into the woods to survive the onslaught of what they perceive as minorities and blacks taking over the country. Rich liberal whites have 'integrated' minorities into the market, but poor whites have been forsaken and remain the archenemies of both.

She was raised by her maternal grandparents until age 8 when her grandfather died, and this was a major cataclysm for her, not only because she had been the apple of her grandfather's eye but because she then went to live with her parents. Up until then, her mother was like a sister who came to visit and was fun to play with.

She lived with her mother first in a trailer park. Her mother was using drugs and alcohol and had different lovers; she ran away to her father's house. Her father lived with no plumbing, electricity, or hot water, with only an outhouse for a bathroom.

Her father would try to discipline her in rather crude ways, telling her she was stupid and trying to enforce gender roles. This problem had a prior history where we see the emergence of the *objet a*. With her grandparents, her grandmother was in charge of discipline, and the grandfather was the loving 'grandmotherly' type in her eyes. Her grandmother caught her peeing standing up repeatedly as her favorite form and insisted that she had to pee sitting down as girls do. She also liked to wear men's underwear and men's shoes, almost military boots. The father continued with this and in addition he told her that she was a woman and explained how men and women have sex, and that she had a vagina and men would put their penis inside her. So she hated penetration, which she experienced as getting fucked over. Her urinary flow was her favorite object (tells jokes) and she disliked her vagina, which she identified with the total body of her mother, whom she regarded as ugly, fat, smelly white trash.

Her favorite form of sex was anal sex, and she liked to penetrate both sexes anally as well as receive anal penetration. From the back or anally there is no sexual difference.

Let me quote you some of her speech:

> As soon as I see him, I know I'll do dirty things to him. We make out in public and then go back to his place where I proceed to ravish him. No one has ever eaten out his asshole. He loves it and is terrified. I know the way I'm touching him is the way that men are supposed to touch women, and I know, because I know, that men say they want this, like this, and then, faced with it, they don't. But I can't help myself. I can't be someone else. Not now, not here. I just want to consume his body, him. He tells me he's never been with someone like me. Like what? I ask. Like a real woman, he tells me. What does that mean? I ask. Someone who knows what she wants, who does what she wants. In almost the same breath, he tells me that he's supposed to be the man, that I'm being the man, that he feels like a girl. It comes up again and again. The way I eat his asshole is like the way he eats pussy. The way he moans is the way he makes women moan when it does that to them. I find all of this incredibly sexy and he finds it terrifying. Exciting, pleasurable, but terrifying, maybe painful. Enjoyable?
>
> Even though this is sex for me, with no future in sight, no commitment, there is still something so serious about it, something so not-casual, despite the circumstances. I could never do this with more than one person at a time. I'm giving him too much of myself. I give too much of myself when I do this.

We say that men conflate sex and love, and that women know, on the contrary, that love is in language, discourse, and speech. This is why women have to talk so much about sex and love and men do not.

> These things I do with my body, with my mouth and my hands, they say something, but they seem to say something that I can't say in language. The sexual drive in the Real is outside language.

> I've been thinking about the lover she had when she started analysis and about his withdrawal, wondering, again, why I do this to myself. He says it's work that is keeping him away, but I'm sure it's not. I'm also not sure, which is what makes things so difficult. I hate not knowing.

Then she met her current boyfriend. Before meeting him, she was fantasizing about planning her future to live with a girlfriend who was also bisexual and androgynous, because she did not believe in commitments or long-term relationships or commitments with men, something she considered stupid and conventional.

Her current boyfriend broke up with his girlfriend, and she was not that into him.

She likes him but is not symptomatic (laughs). She knows who she is and does not want to be seen with him; he is balding, dorky, and nerdy; he feels inferior to her; she is critical and smarter than him; and she knows what she is talking about and has her shit together. She sees herself as a 'whole' person. 'Whole' here is a euphemism. She ends up being confrontational because he is boring and does not self-reflect. 'What is the less favorite thing about me? I don't do relationships; you won't lock me down'.

"I like him, but I don't feel overly liking him. He is not annoying. She is neither in love nor annoyed. Neither of those ways. It's nice, fine'. Then she asked him, 'Do you want to come to my parents for Xmas?'

'I like my mother seeing me be normal or in a relationship. She is seeing me with boyfriend in a way that does not correspond with my reality. Mother's apprehension of the relationship matters'.

She says that her relationship with men fall into two categories: felt rejected and humiliated more like her father versus men that spoil her like her grandfather. She stalks men who are like her grandfather. 'They look dorky, not cool, disgusting, I could do better than him'. She is embarrassed. The bad boy, haughty, asshole – she likes to conquer them, more like her dad. What they have that she wants that gets displaced into being bad asshole. Other types are the tattooed, cool, and married. Someone she should be seen with. Her boyfriend is damaged, aloof, unavailable.

She thinks that she is better than her boyfriend: cooler, smarter, better looking, a come-up for him, he knows that. 'Don't you feel better about yourself now that I desire you'. She does not feel a need for him. With the other men, she cannot get her hands off them. When she is sucking dick and eat their assholes, she sees herself degrading herself.

'I am too good to be doing these things with somebody like Grandfather'. She feels conflicted because he is a good person. She is enjoying having sex with boyfriend. She loves rubbing and sucking dick. She should not do it because he is not good enough. It is pretty knotty, naughty. Dirty, slutty. She had a dream that she was in a football game, responsible for the balls, and scores a touchdown; then she was called by her name.

Associations: She likes watching football; it brings out violence. She does not like her name. Mom wanted to name her Elizabeth. C-section. Hard labor. Her father named her while mother had 24 hours of labor.

She does not know why her name. Her mother still calls her Elizabeth. She remembers hating her name at age 11. She doesn't feel like a man or woman. She does not like either name.

She does not like the way they sound. Her first name is harsh. She hates her last name. With her cats, she refers to herself in the third person. Her name is a common name. Her father's grandmother and his sister have that name.

She is in charge of the balls and scores a touchstone. She does not like cheerleaders. She would have preferred an androgynous name used by both men and women. It is a rejection of father.

In a dream, she is preparing to get raped. A guy gives her lubricant and says this big brutal guy will come in and rape her and hurt her with a big penis. she prepares herself for rape, prepares herself for the pain. She starts masturbating so she is loose and wet.

Associations

Fantasy about a big guy. Fat and muscular. He tattoos her and she gets turned on with the pressing on her body. She is the sexy one, is or has the phallus, and they are weak and disgusting and subordinate. They give her head. Or she is nothing and they are a big penis using her as a sexual object. Or she identifies with the big fat penis or imaginary phallus and she is the one raping a guy in the ass. Or she masturbates to porn where she is both the woman getting raped and the man doing the raping.

Heterosexual intercourse is either women getting raped by men treated as a sexual object, which she does not enjoy intercourse, or she masturbates to porn in which women are getting raped, and she gives herself her own orgasm. She could only have a clitorial orgasm and only if she stimulated herself during sex.

Her current boyfriend, to whom she became quite attached and developed a desire for a long-term relationship with him, did not like anal sex and did not want to be penetrated, resulting in a loss of jouissance for her, but the relationship became more important, and she had to come to terms with the lack of sexual rapport. She came to enjoy vaginal sex, although the jouissance was not as intense, and she let him stimulate her clitoris, although she preferred to do it herself and so did he.

Anorexic Symptom

She is a ribbon in a dream, her fragmented body, me turning small, floating away, disappearing, being chased after by a man. 'I have starved myself. I can feel it in my body, my electrolytes off, my head in a vice, on the verge of losing consciousness when I stand up. But I'm not really losing weight. I'm still a cow. Maybe'.

She reported this initially in relationship to a dream but then never brought it again and did not seem to have a problem with it or with her weight. Then she went to Korea, attended a conference on anorexia, and began talking about it.

Despite her identification with masculinity, she said she idealized petite hyperfeminine and submissive women. She admired and rejected the stereotypically feminine women: 'I can't be it and don't want to be it'. She has a perceived lack of femininity within herself that she idealizes in the Other, and at the same time rejects for herself.

She began starving herself and losing weight, and she looked emaciated and had a cadaveric face like a concentration camp survivor. She did not report it as a problem and resisted seeing it as such. I focused on her interest in anorexia and going to a conference. She acknowledged always touching her bones, a protruding bone. I had her associate to the protruding bone, and she came up with a boner as a metaphor for imaginary phallus. I tell her this is a woman's way to be a man.

She was losing awareness of crossing the line into death. She enjoyed it; it was a high, her anorexic jouissance for the nothing. I expressed concern about the risk that this could lead her into death. As a result of my concern, she began weighing herself and established a limit for her weight despite the deadly enjoyment.

Shoes

Eventually she disclosed that despite her preference for men's shoes, she had five trunks full of women's shoes. She was not satisfied with men's shoes and had a desire for women's shoes but could not wear them and was not comfortable in them; they felt like a simulacrum rather than a masquerade. We remember that *Oedipus* in Greek means 'swollen foot'. I told her that she was trying to discover what is a woman and that neither a man or the simulacrum of a woman satisfied the question and suggested that she could leave it undefined and empty and merely in the form of a question without an answer. (For the record, *swollen* in Sanskrit means 'empty', therefore the emptiness of Oedipus). She was happy with this and began using a feminine version of basketball shoes now made trendy for women as well as flats with flat or low heels.

Termination

She finished her dissertation and her PhD but lost her insurance and could not afford the fee by herself. She was able to get a job as an academic, something that is not easy in the US, to say the least, but that does not start for another six months. We observe here the relationship between the traversal of the fantasy or the fall of the *objet a* and the changes in love and work that Freud considered sufficient criteria for the aim/end of the analysis.

I subjectively would have preferred for the analysis to end once her professional practice as an academic was consolidated. But in fact, Lacan says the analyst ends the session but the analysand ends the analysis. Now she is a disciple of her symptom and the work with the sinthome continues post-termination and has post-termination effects. She had enough of me and the analysis, and I agreed.

The analysis was difficult for her because her symptoms were lodged in character traits that were egosyntonic. I systematically always explored the symptoms in relationship to her character traits, and this was not pleasant for her, but she stuck to it. She bore what was unbearable about analysis. I systematically never gave her any room to regard her symptoms as a problem for me but not for her, with the exception perhaps of the risk of death due to anorexia. In analysis you cannot analyze a symptom, as a psychoanalytic symptom, without first clarifying the subjective position in relationship to the symptom as a form of jouissance. We never take for granted that the symptom is a problem, however painful, although we at first strategically pretend this to be the case. We tacitly know that the analysand is in love with their symptoms and the symptom is how the analysand 'makes out' with the Unconscious, as Lacan says in RSI.

Because the analysis was painful, or open-heart surgery, she never expressed much regret for losing me. I decided to make a mistake on purpose, following what Harari taught me that an analyst is established by their mistakes in the Freudian sense of parapraxis, I simply said once that I would miss our work together so that I would remain as a pure desire and an acceptance of lack, no longer an imaginary object, whether idealized or persecutory, and an object that she could discard. It was true, however, and not make-believe; otherwise, I would not have said it.

Conclusion

Are there any structured signifiers that are universal or common to most people? This is what Freud's biographer, Ernest Jones (1916), argued. Here, Lacanian signifiers are equivalent to Jungian archetypes. Archetypes, for Jung, although images, were symbolic elements equivalent to genes.

The signifiers for the cases were: virgin, gigolo, hole, staff, symbols, castration, phallic woman, authority, father, big Other, son, mother, doctor, sinner, man, 'fucker', snake, parricide, bohemian, woman, sinner, girl as a scholar, feminine jouissance, mystic jouissance, peachy, little devil, special boy, fallen angel, and mystical jouissance.

The signifiers are the Real pieces that fell off the structure and that operate in reality, rather than the other way around. It is not that the structure operates in reality and the pieces fall away into oblivion. The structure is invisible and does not operate in reality; only the Real pieces do.

What do I mean by 'Real structure'? I refer to the oedipal structure that is no longer Symbolic as Lacan said. Lacan said that the Oedipus complex was a dream of Freud, and I would add, represents a mathematical structure. Oedipus is Real as a mathematical structure, and virtual as a dream, or fiction. The pure mother is a virgin, the obedient boy could be used as a gigolo by sacred or secular authorities. He contains the hole of the vagina in the anus. The mother represents the lack of the Other. The complete mother is the phallic mother who has the pants in the house. Now she can wear the pants either because she stole the pants from the father or because the father gave them to her.

The father represents the values of the culture and ancestors. The doctor is holy, like women, while men are sinners and fornicators/*masterbators*. Are girls undisciplined, as Freud said, 'They have no superego', or are girls more disciplined in school? In any case, a scholar girl is something special, and if you are special enough, you will find her in a library lane riding a white pony and selecting her favorite books. The girl in the white pony is Athena emerging from inside her father's head or, at least, from the bosom of his storehouse memory.

Are children pure or perverse? Children have no fixed ego, so they are not perverse. There is no difference between a child's purity and the mystic jouissance of the beginner's mind. The end is like the beginning, and after having gone through the childishness and horror of unconscious fantasy and polymorphous perversion, the analysand goes back to being a child with mature and wise characteristics.

The capacity for sublimation is a drive that I measure with imaginary numbers. One can also acquire higher levels of sublimation ascending the y- (i-) imaginary axis. The lessening of symptoms increases the potential for sublimation, making more energy available for other uses. However, I acknowledge that assessing the capacity for sublimation is an intuitive and conceptual axiom that does not have to be proven in science. It depends on interests, capacities, and creative activities. However, a more precise instrument could also be developed.

To conclude, I offer a table of the signifiers shared by all subjects in this book. This is not a representative sample in the statistical sense but a representative sample of norms established not by statistics but by normative society. I note that anxiety is a more common symptom than depression. I can conclude that the hypothesis advanced by many is true. The 21st century is a century not of depression, but of anxiety, the result of 'too much' rather than not enough: encore. The 20th century was the century of two World Wars: impermanence, death, and loss.

Case of M	Martin	Chinese	S	Literary Benevolence	Case of J
Failure of identification with father	Desire to kill father	Refusal of father	My son the doctor	My son the brilliant scholar	His phallus is the name of his kabbalistic father in the transference
Special to mother	Special to mother	Special to mother	Special to mother	Special to mother	
Anxiety depersonalization		anxiety addiction	anxiety irritability	anxiety Depression	Anxiety grief
Case of M	Martin		Chinese	S	Literary Benevolence
Failure of identification with father	Desire to kill father		Refusal of father	My son the doctor	My son the brilliant scholar
Special to mother	Special to mother		Special to mother	Special to mother	Special to mother
Anxiety depersonalization	Anxiety Addiction		anxiety irritability	anxiety depression	

A positive response to treatment is represented by a decrease of *x* numbers and an increase of i numbers. Higher levels of sublimation predict better outcomes, and the capacity for sublimation can be increased in a virtuous cycle (indicated by prime numbers). Sublimation is not a socialized ego drive, but an evolved form of jouissance. The ego is useful as a concept to understand narcissism. The reality principle is a principle of the subject. The concept of self can be used for either undifferentiated or recognizable self-experience.

Finally, if we plot all the complex numbers on a complex plane, we find that posttreatment all the numbers are on the right-side imaginary side of the graph. How do we obtain imaginary complex numbers that are both golden and imaginary? And how does this relate to the question of the phallus, which for Lacan was equivalent to the golden number, and how does the golden number 1.684 (a symbolic phallus: $\Phi \rightarrow -\left(\sqrt{1}\right)$ in a quadratic equation transforms into an imaginary number and a different form of jouissance? Phi transforms into i or $(\sqrt{-1})$. The 1.68 includes infinitesimals while the imaginary number is a negative unit that cannot be subdivided further.

> Mathematically Phi – phi (1,618 – 0,618) = 1. This can be seen as the formula for the phallic function of castration. Phi – phi = the "symbolic phallus" minus the 'imaginary phallus' . . . −phi or the lack of the imaginary phallus generates a lack-of-being; a hole within the whole that subjects endlessly try to fill with objets a. It does not work because -phi is a signifier without a signified (phallic function). It is a symbolic castration that creates a gap thereby representing a point of lack in the subject.
>
> (Moncayo and Romanowicz, 2015, p. 130)

Phi − phi = 1 is the formula for symbolic castration, where only by accepting the lack (−phi) with the help of Phi can the subject arrive at One as an imaginary number or i (imaginary in the mathematical, not Lacanian, sense). Otherwise, the subject keeps looking for the fantasy object in reality and in the axis of real numbers (real in the mathematical sense and in the sense of external reality).

According to the formula Phi – phi, as the formula for symbolic castration, Phi subtracts the a (phi) and turns every i(a) and i (a′1, 2, 3, 4) into a 1 that can be used as either a real or imaginary number. Phi is the quantity or power by which phi changes into 1 as either a series of real numbers or a series of imaginary numbers. In this sense, the formula for castration also qualifies as a logarithm for images.

By phi missing from Phi, Phi becomes either a real 1 or an imaginary 1. One has the *objet a* missing from it. With a or -a missing in real whole-body images, the subject tries to fill the hole with other alter egos and their missing *objet a* in a futile exercise that is played at the level of images. Instead of another whole image or number, what needs to be symbolized and made manifest in numbers is the 1 as an imaginary number that appears in the hole in the image. Otherwise, the alleged whole objects and alter egos or intersubjective others go from being whole numbers to being like the song of Ricky Martin: 'a little bit of Monica, Gloria, and Veronica in my life,' the partial *objet a* of the subject in its various iterations.

Plotnitsky (2009) has quoted Leibniz in this regard: 'Imaginary roots are a subtle and wonderful resort of the divine spirit, a kind of hermaphrodite between existence and non-existence (inter En and non Ens Amphibio).'

> [T]he square root of −1 does not correspond to anything that is subject to our intuition, anything real-in the mathematical sense of the term – and yet it must be conserved, along with its full functioning.
>
> (Lacan, 1975–1976a, p. 29)

The phallus is a missing or non-existing object/signifier and a signifier without a signified (Ø) and in this sense bears a resemblance to the existence/nonexistence of imaginary numbers as well as to the mark of the unmarked.

The bracket on the zero is 1 but leaves the zero intact as a concept and a number. The bar instead makes the zero a no concept, a no number, a no name, and an empty space.

Within Lacanian psychoanalysis the barred zero is a pure form of the negative that is not a point in space in the sense of an object but simply a symbolic empty place of substitution and movement for representations. It is in this sense that Lacan says that the symbolic phallus appears in the place of the signifier of a lack or the lack of a signifier. This is even though the symbolic phallus as Capital Phi is also a Golden number within the axis of real numbers.

Within the symbolic function of Capital Phi, small +phi and −phi represent the presence and absence of substitutive and imaginary signifiers for the phallus. But why then does Lacan use the square root of −1 as a signifier for the phallus that is an imaginary number and not a real number like the golden number?

$\sqrt{-1}$ is an impossible number: there is no square root of −1. Yet we are using it in calculations in mathematics and physics all the time. In the same way although the phallus as such may not exist (impossible to represent) it may also lead to true conclusions regarding certain forms of phenomena described by psychoanalysis.

Imaginary numbers may be considered impossible, yet they follow all the basic rules of mathematics like addition, subtraction, and multiplication. In addition, the unit imaginary number, i, has the property of cycling through four different values of multiplication, as shown:

$$i^1 = i$$
$$i^2 = -1$$
$$i^3 = -i$$
$$i^4 = 1$$

$$i^5 = i \times i^4 = i$$
$$i^6 = i^2 \times i^4 = -i$$
$$i^7 = i^3 \times i^4 = -i$$
$$i^8 = i^4 \times i^4 = 1$$

The cycling of i yields four terms: i, −1, −i, and 1.

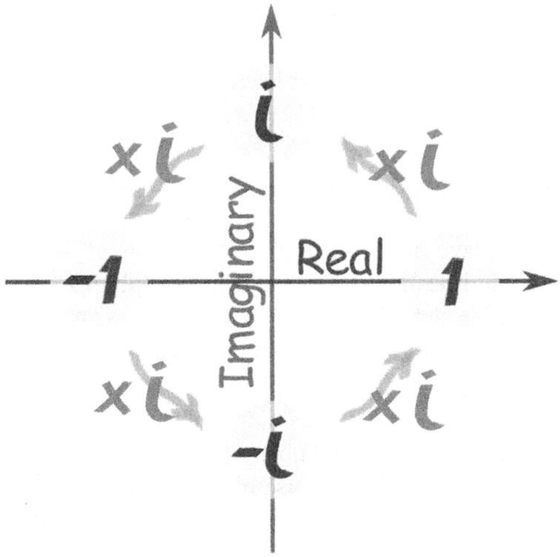

The neutral point between 1 and −1 and i and −i represents the center of two axis: the imaginary and real axes. The Imaginary can be the fantasy of the imagination (archetype), rather than the Imaginary. For example, the Nazis used the swastika symbol of Buddhist origins and perverted it with an imaginary meaning. The imagination is based on the poetics of metaphor and resemblance, and reveals the glory of emptiness, the consummated nature. The real axis is never Real. It consists of our drives and fixations that need to be sublated not by the Imaginary but by the imagination.

In the graph there is a circle that combines both axes: i, −1, −i, 1. From this circle, we can extend a wave of water, or a target, for example, to 2i, −2, −2i, 2, 2i, and so on. This represents Buddhism as a series of circles within circles, with the teaching representing the particles, and the waves representing the experience of jouissance/meditation.

I can understand numbers as quantum particles and not only as numbers that are part of a symbolic system laid on top of ontology and the Real of the things themselves. Instead, imaginary numbers are the things in themselves as particles, not as waves as waves numbers remain outside the symbolic system. The Real is a series of quantum waves in the emptiness of the vacuum that are perceived as the forms of matter (the visual world is a simulation).

Quantum waves are Real energy outside the Symbolic system that is measured with nontrivial zeros in the 0.5 critical line. You have waves starting at zero and expanding outwardly to 2 to 4 with phase space-time being the space in-between diacritical numbers indicated by the arrows. $0 \rightarrow 2 \rightarrow 4 \rightarrow$ etc. We can visualize how the waves irradiate from a point 0 that does not exist: 0, 1, 2, 3, and so on.

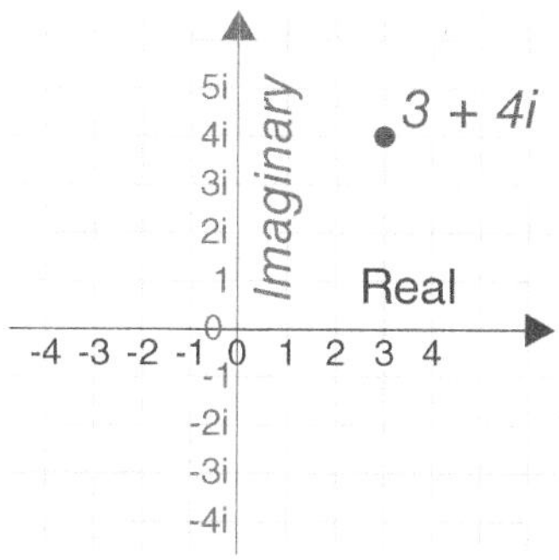

https://www.mathsisfun.com/algebra/complex-plane.html accessed March 5, 2023.

Before we proceed further, we need to clarify certain similarities and differences between mathematical and Lacanian terms. The use of imaginary numbers in mathematics differs from the concept of the Imaginary in Lacan. Images in the sense of the Imaginary have no diacritical numbers unless we reduce color to number. For this reason, imaginary numbers in a Lacanian sense are Symbolic. By the same reasoning real numbers in the mathematical sense are not Real in the Lacanian use of the term.

Lacan talks about the phallus in several ways throughout his work.

1. Lacan writes about the imaginary phallus as 1 and −1 in real axis.
2. He also speaks about the imaginary phallus and the *objet a* in terms of the golden number proportion 0.618.
3. The phallus is also described as i number ($\sqrt{-1}$).

Using 1 and −1 is a very crude way of talking about the phallus as animal imaginary genital jouissance without signifiers. With speaking beings and language, phi and –phi is dependent on castration that assigns them their place.

Lacan said that the null set or the signifier of a symbolic lack is related to the Capital Phi or the symbolic phallus, which is an absence and is equivalent to symbolic castration and does not have the positive and negative signs that Lacan ascribes to the imaginary phallus as phi and −phi. It is the symbolic phallus that gives access to phallic jouissance. Without castration, there is no phallic jouissance, properly speaking; there may be copulation or rape but no phallic jouissance.

But ultimately the phallus does not exist and to experience this void, or the phallus that does not exist as the no signified, may be traumatic.

The subject needs the name as the symbolic phallus (Phi) that substitute for the imaginary phallus (−phi). Then from the name that is meaningless or is a “no name” or simply “this” the experience of the void as the Other jouissance is possible.

Lacan says that a name brings a relative stop to the sliding of signifiers and to the production of a new imaginary *objet a*. But the signifier of a lack in the Other is the name of the nameless or is the name that points to an absence that is also a presence in the Real. This is where the name also links to the Real face of the *objet a* as the index of a void of presence and an Other jouissance not-all under the phallic function, for which feminine jouissance is one of its forms. This is what the square root of -1 represents, in our opinion.

The symbolic phallus moves the subject in the direction of the square root of -1 because it does not exist and has no direct reference to the penis. In 1973, Lacan stated that the symbolic phallus is ‘the signifier which does not have a signified’ (Seminar XX, 1972–1973, p. 75). The square root of -1 is a special signifier without a signified or better a number without a number.

The statement that the symbolic phallus or F appears in the place of the lack of the signifier in the Other, seems to link the F and the lack in the Other, the symbol of which is the same symbol as the null or empty set (Ø). Lacan uses the math symbol for the null set for the signifier of a lack in the Other.

$\emptyset \rightarrow \Phi \rightarrow \sqrt{-1}$ (Formula adapted by Miller, 2015)

The Lack in the Other (Ø) transforms into Phi (Φ) and into $\sqrt{-1}$. The $\sqrt{-1}$ is outside phallic jouissance. The missing signifier transforms into a structure with a missing piece that transforms into symbolic wholeness in emptiness (a unary negation). The law and the structure do not exist or dissipate, yet they generate the order of the structure. The law is ultimately the Law of Wu, as a unary negation. The mystery is how the law of emptiness (Kong) transforms into the Taoist and Confucian virtues of particularity and propriety.

$$(\Phi \rightarrow -\sqrt{-1})$$

$$(-\sqrt{-1} \rightarrow \Phi)$$

Phallic jouissance can go beyond phallic jouissance and become the third jouissance, the third jouissance can go back to the second, and the second go back to the first. Mathematically Phi – phi (1,618–0,618) = 1. This can be seen as the formula for the phallic function of castration. Phi – phi = the ‘symbolic phallus’ minus the ‘imaginary phallus’. The First jouissance represents the bad infinity of metonymy and displacement of representations.

Negative phi or the lack of the imaginary phallus generates a lack-of-being, a hole within the whole that subjects endlessly try to fill with *objet a*. It does not work because -phi is a signifier without signified (phallic function). It is a symbolic castration that creates a gap, thereby representing a point of lack in the subject.

A positive response to treatment is represented by a decrease of x numbers and an increase in the y-axis, or i numbers. 'Higher levels of sublimation predict better outcomes, and the capacity for sublimation can be increased in a virtuous cycle (indicated by prime numbers)' (above) and at the same time the sublime number ($\sqrt{-1}$) goes back into phallic jouissance. The sublime number refers to the quantification of events: art, religion, scholarship, exercise, martial culture, music, and the like.

Cases also retain numbers on the bottom-right quadrant of imaginary numbers. This means that the tree of knowledge not only ascends to the heights but also descends with deep roots inside the earth. In a case with a history of addiction, the subject remains prone to addiction within sobriety. This means that the subject remains prone to speak of the Real without words, or with mathematics. These are the numbers in a binary matrix that represent the character and analysis of the subject.

1. Chinese Unconscious

$$\begin{pmatrix} 2 & -2i \\ 2i & 2 \end{pmatrix}$$

$$(2+-2\mathrm{i})\times(2\mathrm{i}+2)(4+4\mathrm{i})$$

2. Case of S

$$\begin{pmatrix} 1 & -2i \\ 2i & 1 \end{pmatrix}$$

$$(1+-2\mathrm{i})\times(2\mathrm{i}+1)(2+4\mathrm{i})$$

3. Case of Martin

$$\begin{pmatrix} 3 & -2i \\ -2i & 3 \end{pmatrix}$$

$$(3+-2\mathrm{i})\times(-2\mathrm{i}+3)\rightarrow(6+-4\mathrm{i})$$

$$\begin{pmatrix} 2 & -5i \\ -5i & 2 \end{pmatrix}$$

$$(2+-5\mathrm{i})\times(-5\mathrm{i}+2)\rightarrow 4+10\mathrm{i})$$

4. Literary Benevolence

$$\begin{pmatrix} 0 & -7i \\ -7i & 0 \end{pmatrix}$$

$$(0+-7)\times(-7+0)\rightarrow(0+-14\text{i})$$

5. Case of M

$$\begin{pmatrix} 2 & 4i \\ 4i & 2 \end{pmatrix}$$

$$(2+4\text{i})\times(4\text{i}+2)\rightarrow(4+8\text{i})$$

Appendix I

Standard Proven Probability that a Pair of Cards Could be of the Same Color (Same Quality X)

This experiment has an intuitive adhesion that makes it immediately comprehensible. In the past, before writing this book, I desisted from detailing a case history in psychoanalysis given that today a release of confidentiality is required to present personal findings and that this could prove to be deleterious, harmful, or undermine the positive post-analytical results of an analysis for a subject. This is despite the fact that Freud's ethics assigned more importance to the advancement of science than to concerns about confidentiality. I have never revealed details of cases who have asked me not to reveal anything about their case in published writing. The details of their case helped me strengthen the theory, and the theory helped me illuminate the enigmas of speech, so then it could be generalized to other cases. In the past, I limited myself to vignettes.

One morning I awoke early to find this entire experiment flowing from my fingers in a single sitting. Because I am a layperson, definitely not a specialized mathematician, and having no reason under critical or practical reason to cling to falsehood, however unfortunate or beneficial a surprising discovery may be, I welcome specialists to falsify or support my results.

How do you solve for the standard probability? How do we obtain a positive significance versus results that are not significant? 1 versus 0 or both, versus 0.5: the critical line where nontrivial zeros appear. Trivial zeros are nonsignificant. One represents significance, and 0 is trivial nonsignificance. However, 0 can also represent emptiness and nontriviality.

First, I want to make explicit that in this experiment the color of the card is equivalent to electron charges, as a step-by-step parallel process. We are studying the behavior of cards as a metaphor or analogy for the behavior of electrons. In the same way, the logic of the cards can be transferred to the logic of the psyche.

In science, the first experiment is seen as scientific, while for psychology, it is considered an unscientific projection from animate humans to inanimate subatomic particles.

Two cards are drawn, without replacement, from a standard 52-card deck. Find the probability that both cards are the same color. Color here is equivalent to identical positive or negative charges in electrons. I could also extend this unit to the signifier. Would this lead to negative colors and positive colors, dark or light? What is the color rather than the sound of the signifier? Conversely, sounds can be seen as color. A sunset scene is teeming with signifiers and signification.

Matching polarization is equivalent to having the equivalent color.

Pick a color: 2 ways.

Each deck has 26 cards.

For picking the first card, we have 26 ways since 52/2 = 26.

When we have picked the first card, then there are 25 cards and ways left.

Answer by Fombitz (32,378) at www.algebra.com

Pick two cards without replacement: 26C2 = (26 × 25)/(1 × 2) = 325

Pick two cards randomly: 52C2

P (2 cards same color): (2 × 325)/(52C2) = 0.4902

Answer by Fombitz (32378) at www.algebra.com

$$P(R) = \frac{26}{52} = \frac{1}{2}$$

1st Red:

$$P(R) = \frac{25}{51}$$

2nd Red:

$$P(R, \quad R) = \left(\frac{1}{2}\right) \times \left(\frac{25}{51}\right)$$

$$P(R, \quad R) = \frac{25}{102}$$

Because there are the same number of reds and blacks,

$$P(B, \quad B) = \frac{25}{102} \cdot$$

The probability that the cards are the same color is

$$P = P(R, \quad R) + P(B, \quad B)$$

$$P = \frac{25}{102} = \frac{25}{102}$$

$$P = \frac{25}{51} = 0.4902 \cdot$$

The result of the standard probability for a pair of cards to be the same or different color is low or insignificant. There is a low insignificant probability (0) that a pair of cards will be of the same color (1).

Experiment

In an experiment using not only 2 but also 11 pairs, randomly selected cards (out of a deck of 52 cards) are dealt facedown. Once a pair is laid facedown on the table, the rules for interpreting the results are stated: same color wins; different color loses.

For example, for the first deal of cards, out of 11 random pairs there were 8 random wins and 3 loses.

What are the 8-to-3 odds of winning if the same color wins?

Probability of

Winning = (0.7273) or 72.72%
Losing = (0.2727) or 27.27%

"Odds for" winning: 8:3

"Odds against" winning: 3:8

First Set: same color wins, different color loses.

1. First try.
   WIN (72% chance of winning, simply by selecting the rules)
2. Second random trial: same color wins, different color loses
   Same results in reverse: 3 wins, 8 losses.
   LOSS (7 or 72% chance of losing)
   Third random trial same color wins, different color loses.
   3 wins, 8 losses.
   LOSS
   (one win/two losses)
   72% chance of either winning or losing according to house rules. Regardless of a win or lose outcome, the pattern is preserved. 1 win, 2 loses.
   Second set with opposite rules: different color wins, same color loses.
   First Trial: same color loses, different color wins.
   6 pairs of different colors/5 pairs of same color
   WIN (66% chance of winning).
   Second Trial Run: same color loses, different color wins.
   6 pairs of different colors; 5 of same
   WIN (66% chance of winning)
   Third Trial Run: Same color loses, different color wins.

7 same color/ 4 different color
LOSS (chance of losing = 64%)
Second Set Results: 2 wins/1 loss

This pattern is not happening by chance; the pattern is a tripartite structure. Chance or automaton works within a determinate structure. Chance only looks like chance because, as Einstein said, G-d actually does not play dice with the universe. Probability is only apparent randomness. Behind the large cardinal micro numbers lies a macro pattern of only four numbers. Zero and 1 are present in all units, while 3 is the structure that mediates between 0, 1, and 2. Four is what binds them together to hold the larger set of cardinal numbers, as if it were a handle for G-d's hand to manage the galaxies (only a metaphor but the handle may be dark matter) or there in another galaxy behind the observable one, holding the visible 1 together.

These are the rules:

Either the same color wins and a different color loses or a different color wins and the same color loses.

Once the rules are stated an interactive pattern emerges between the two cards (properties are interdependent, or their differences and similarities arise together). Two cards could also represent a pair of subatomic particles, or two coins. In fact, physicists have no problem in establishing equivalence between two cards, two coins, two subatomic particles, or subjects, on their way to theorizing. The axioms do not have to be proven, thank goodness.

The results for the two cards are created together when cards are presented together facedown. When an observer looks at reality according to certain rules, or when you define reality according to rules, then reality of both cards is summoned together. Red and black do not exist until you turn them over. One of the follow-up questions that I have from the experiment is whether two particles will always be the opposite of what the rules indicated, or what is the pattern or frequency of this opposition.

Repeated trial runs are automaton or false chance in Aristoteles, while the pattern according to structure is true chance or what Aristoteles called Tyche.

In groups of three sets of repeated trial runs according to the rules, the probability is either very significant (0.7 or 0.8) or very insignificant by the same ratio. What interests us is not the statistical significance or insignificance of the probability but explaining the fact that in either case, the ratio is the same with the opposite sign. This is a structural pattern, and how does this structure emerge?

In the two sets of three trials, rules can either win twice and lose once or lose twice and win once. Sometimes phenomena comply with the rule grid not once but twice, but the third time it does not, as well as vice versa. Nature, randomness, or the Real seems to support difference more than sameness, so it responds affirmatively more often to rules that emphasize difference. As soon as a natural thing is exposed to thought, it can be identified as difference 2 out of 3 times and 1 in 3 times by sameness. At least 1 in 3 times the rules of difference fail, or nature opposes them, meaning that there is a 1 in 3 chance that phenomena or the Real will not follow the rules of difference and a 2 in 3 chance that it will. Regarding the rules of sameness, there is a 1 in 3 chance that the Real will follow them, while 2 in 3 times it will not.

The practical consequence of the logic of the experiment, and the structure or pattern that emerges from it, solves a problem of Lacanian theory that I was not able to solve otherwise for my book on Seminar XXIII. The question was as follows. In Seminar XXIII, Lacan argues that it is the Real rather than the Symbolic that ties the knot of four together. The Real becomes the Third rather than the Symbolic. The third now becomes the Real of the third jouissance instead of the third of the treasury of the signifier. This was a new logic proposed for the knot of four. I use one of the knots of four Lacan uses in Seminar XXIII. Extrapolation in this case has to do with the dimensions you can count on one hand. It has the same meaning in an abstract knot and in four dimensions of experience.

Lacan postulated a new knot of four that included a fourth ring that he associated with the sinthome as a new form of the name of the father that comes out of the Real. The new knot of three needs to be undone and retied with the help of a fourth ring coming out of the third of the Real. So why does Lacan say that the fourth ring comes out of the Real?

The experiment provides an answer to this question. The sinthome or the NoF comes out of the Real rather than from the Symbolic or the Imaginary because the Real as the Third is self-same, while the Imaginary and the Symbolic cannot exist without each other. The Real also emerges from the knot but remains outside the Symbolic and the Imaginary.

The experiment shows that although 2 out of 3 times, difference (in images or words) will prevail over sameness, regardless of the rules set by the observer, 1 out of 3 times, the self-same of the undifferentiated plenum of the Real (the Real always returns to the same place), will prevail over difference. When the Real is taken as zero rather than 1, or a 1 that includes zero, then the third becomes a fourth (instead of 1, 2, 3, we have four elements: 0, 1, 2, 3).

Psychically rules are Symbolic and follow from either rationality or the superego. "Do it because I say so whether apparently logical or not". If the ego/superego, or the repressive unconscious, seek sameness with the One of ideals (Imaginary) to repress difference, then 2 out of 3 times, the Real of the drive will oppose the superego. The One of the Real opposes the One of the Imaginary. Although the signifier is linked to difference, the drive as jouissance is linked to the sameness of jouissance in its three levels. Repression fails 1 out of 3 times. If the ego/superego seeks a difference from the drive, then 1 out of 3 times, nature, or the Real of the drive will respond with sameness.

In Freudian Lacanian theory, as outlined in the book, there are three psychical systems and three registers of experience (Ucs.Pcs./Pcs.Cs./Pcpt.Cs and RSI). Are these systems/dimensions correlated with the two rules and the three responses to each rule?

When the rule/observer expects sameness from phenomena (Nature, Real), then there is a 1 in 3 chance that the Ucs. and Pcpt cs system will perceive in acquiescence of social norms and a 2 in 3 chance that opposition to the rule will be the case. This is consistent with the fact that psychoses and perversions can be defined as various forms of rebellion or disavowal and only neurosis represents avowal or compliance with social norms at the subject's own expense. The return of the repressed has a 2 in 3 chance of taking place, while successful repression takes place 1 out of 3 times.

When the Pcs.cs. rule demands a difference in expression, then there is a 2 in 3 chance that the Pcpt.cs. and Ucs. will respond with difference, and a 1 in 3 chance that they will respond in opposition to the rule of difference and in acquiescence with the rule of sameness. The chances for repression or for expression, in consciousness or the unconscious, or in the two sets are the same. The ratio between the two forces is the same: 1 for repression and 2 for expression or the return of the repressed.

If, for example, the rule is the command to have sex (difference leading to sameness), there is a 2 in 3 chance that the subject of the rule, as its pairwise companion, will dream about having sex, and a 1 in 3 chance that they will not. If the rule is to not have sex, there is a 1 in 3 chance that the subject of the rule will have sex in a dream and 2 in 3 chance that they will not.

In addition, the Cs. and the Ucs. systems are also redoubled in the structure. When this redoubling takes place, the Cs. includes the Pcpt.cs. system and the Pcs.cs. system, and the Unconscious includes the Ucs. proper (repressed Unconscious under primary repression) and the Pcs., which is unconscious in a descriptive sense but can also be suppressed by the Cs. and secondary repression. Because of this structural replication or redoubling, the newly internally differentiated systems can either work together or in opposition to one another.

The conclusion is that rules define beforehand the binary win/lose meaning of a pair or any pair of particles or signifiers (what is weak and what is strong, what is up or down, etc.) Two out of three times house rules lose twice and win once or win twice and lose once. Whatever rules you have to distribute value/meaning in terms of difference or sameness, will define the values of variables 2 out of 3 times.

The next step is to identify images with the Ucs., and words with the Pcs. cs. With the replication of the structure, words and the Pcs.cs. system can also function in the Ucs.Pcs.cs. system, and images can also function in the Pcs.cs. system. Images (Imaginary) will generate repression 1 out of 3 times, and the law in words (Symbolic) will generate opposition 2 out of 3 times. Generating a license for consumption has a 2 in 3 chances of prevailing in images, while repressive authority has a 2 in 3 chances of prevailing in words.

Rules/signifiers are particles; what remains outside is a Real wave that opposes the rules. A wave acquires its characteristics based on the rules, sometimes in images, sometimes in words, sometimes as repression, sometimes as the repressed, depending on the initial definitions. Pairwise organization means either the same or different. Two can be either 1 (same color of two cards) or 2 (different color between two cards), not 1 because it can be 2 and not 2 because it can be 1: not/1–not/2.

For Lacan, the particle/signifier/observation splits the Real thing. The Real withdraws from the signifier and represents a 1 in 3 chance that the phenomenon or thing in question will not be accurately described by the signifying grid and the images superimposed on nature. If the Real is incorporated, and an image/particle/photon/pixel is also a wave, or the signifier is also a signifier of jouissance, then the likelihood that the grid is true increases by 33%.

If the Real is not included in images, words, and things, then objects are only objects in reference to a linguistic grid, including the person observing. When the grid does not include a 1 in 3 uncertainty factor, or impermanent variance, then the symbolic grid becomes the Imaginary. When the grid includes the unknowable wave of jouissance, then the grid is also Real rather than fantasized, and things are particles/signifiers as well as waves. This is the ideal set of conditions that sustains the Universe.

Finally, another example of the patterns described could be found in human relationships between the sexes today, both biologically and psychically. If subjects commit to a partner that at first was loved in the Imaginary, there is a 1 in 3 chance that the partner will be left for a lover and a 2 in 3 chance that the relationship will succeed. If the subject commits to someone they do not first love in the Imaginary, there is a 2 in 3 chance the partner will be left for a lover.

If the subject chooses a lover over a partner who was loved in the Imaginary at the outset of the relationship, there is a 2 in 3 chance the relationship with a lover will succeed. If a lover is chosen over a partner that was not initially loved in the Imaginary, then there is a 2 in 3 chance that the relationship with a lover will succeed and 1 in 3 chance that it will fail.

The 0.7 or 0.3 chance that a relationship will either succeed or fail represents the fact that the margin of variance will contain other moderating or accidental variables such as level of hate, conflicts with in-laws, cultural or religious conflicts, family illnesses, economic hardship, presence, or absence, of children, and so on.

Conclusion

Structural patterns are not happening by chance, because working within probability, particles fulfill the pattern that already is a tripartite structure before the particles existed. Phenomenologically all we see at first is random fluctuations of particles in the void. Chance works within a determinate structure that appears random, but is this chance, or how the subject makes their destiny with the available structure?

In science, this is also called Laplace's demon, which does not need chance or probability because they intuitively know where things are at all times. This is referred to as determinism without any uncertainty. Descartes instead had G-d as the subject supposed to know, which provides a guarantee to the workings of the universe. With quantum mechanics from Einstein onward, and with Heisenberg's uncertainty principle, the universe is no longer entirely known. In medieval theology, the Demiurge, was the equivalent of dark matter as what G-d used (the map, the structure) to build the universe. The creator and the Demiurge are both hidden (dark energy and dark matter). Einstein believed in determinism and a G-d-ordered universe. G-d is uncertain like an axiom, so it is an unknown we can trust like money. It is the same with the law of karma. We can trust that the sun will rise tomorrow and that if we do good work, we will get paid.

One of the follow-up research questions that I have from the experiment is whether two particles will always be the opposite of what the rules indicated, or what is the pattern or frequency of this opposition.

Repeated trial runs are automaton or false chance in Aristoteles, while the pattern according to a slowly evolving structure is true chance, or what Aristoteles called Tyche where structural change takes place. Quantity or the micro does not determine the macro pattern or number, as Gregory Bateson (1979) put it.

> It is impossible, in principle, to explain any pattern by invoking a single quantity. But note that a ratio between two quantities is already the beginning of pattern. In other words, quantity and pattern are of different logical types and do not readily fit together in the same thinking. What appears to be a genesis of a phantom by quantity arises when the pattern was latent before the quantity had impact on the system. The familiar case is that of tension which will break a chain at the weakest link. Under change of a quantity, tension, a latent difference is made manifest or, as the photographers would say, developed. The development of photographic negative is precisely the making manifest of latent differences laid down in the photographic emulsion by previous differential exposure to light.
>
> (p. 58)

Number is different from quantity. This difference is basic for any sort of theorizing in behavioral science, for any sort of imagining of what goes on between organisms, or inside organisms, as part of their thought processes, which may not be like ours. Numbers are the product of counting. Quantities are the product of measurement. This means that numbers can conceivably be accurate because there is a discontinuity between each integer and the next period, between two and three, there is an orbital jump. In the case of quantity, there is no such jump; and because jump is missing in the world of quantity, it is impossible for any quantity to be exact. You can have exactly three tomatoes, but you can never have exactly 3 gallons of water. Always quantity is approximate (idem, Bateson, 1979, p. 53).

The ratio between two numbers is a unit of signification whether in numbers or letters. But the pattern and the symbol do not fit together into a single whole as predicted by Dilthey. When the quantity of heat rises, the pattern of heat was already there before the quantity of heat rose. Numbers or integers require that one is able to count to a pattern of four with a single hand. Patterns or structures are topological, Borromean, and Lacanian, SIR!

The Real is a wave outside (ex-sistence) the particles of existence, the Symbolic is a particle or a hole, and the Imaginary is the consistency of the wave and the particle and the fact that sometimes energy appears to be a particle and sometimes a wave. In this case, the Real is a visible material reality, and reality is an invisible Wave (of dark matter); form is emptiness, and emptiness is form.

Appendix II

The Philosophical and Psychoanalytic Concept of History

History is known as a series of past events that have an intrinsic pattern or structure. Most people refer to history as the next bad thing coming or what you do not want to happen to you. History always returns to the same bad thing. Usually, history documents politics, governments, wars, and change. History also points to the future, insofar as people want to make the future a better place for the new generations.

In psychoanalysis, *history* refers to an individual's past experiences, particularly those from early childhood, which are believed to significantly shape current thoughts, feelings, and actions, and can be accessed and analyzed through the analytic process to understand unconscious desires and structures. Essentially, a person's "psychical history" is considered crucial to understanding a person's present struggles and problems.

The Unconscious in psychoanalysis emphasizes the role of repressed memories and conflicts from early life that continue to impact present behavior, even if the individual is not consciously aware of them. Freud's psychosexual stages of development (oral, anal, phallic, genital, latency) are pivotal in shaping personality and are often examined in psychoanalytic psychotherapy.

Through the analytic process, individuals may reexperience past traumatic events and fantasies, allowing them to process, traverse, and transform these experiences into their current understanding of themselves.

Psychohistory

Psychohistory is a field that applies psychoanalytic theory to analyze historical figures and events, attempting to understand their desires and psychological dynamics based on available information. This is also the field of psychobiography.

Different Views of History

Different philosophers have viewed history in various ways, with some seeing it as a divinely guided process unfolding according to God's plan, while others considered it a progression towards greater human freedom (Hegel, 1822), or a series of repeating cycles of rise and fall (Eliade, 1949; Cassirer, 1946) across different civilizations.

St. Augustine believed history is a linear progression guided by God, culminating in the final judgment, with events like the fall of Adam, the exodus of the Jews, and the life of Jesus as pivotal points.

Georg Wilhelm Friedrich Hegel considered history as a dialectical process moving toward realizing human freedom, with each stage containing contradictions that lead to a higher synthesis.

The general views are discussed next.

Teleological View

Many philosophers, particularly religious thinkers, believed history has a purpose or goal, often tied to divine providence.

Cyclical View

Some philosophers saw history as a series of repeating patterns, with civilizations rising and falling in similar ways. History, in this view, must strive to return or repeat the sacred origin of humanity. The second order of instinct tends toward the life of reproduction, led by the chaos of nature. Civilizations are destroyed by this chaos. History is not only the repetition of progress but the same repetition of the same problems.

Linear View

Enlightenment thinkers often saw history as a continuous progression toward greater human advancement.

Hegel's (1830) philosophy of history emphasizes the development of freedom and the consciousness of freedom over the course of world history. For Hegel (1770–1831), this development is marked by conflict and struggle, rather than smooth uninterrupted progress, and is manifested for the most part in political developments construed broadly, including world-historical events such as the French Revolution and in the significant actions of world-historical "heroes" such as Alexander the Great, Napoleon Bonaparte, George Washington, and Winston Churchill, and in the achievements of peoples and nations.

According to Hegel, the end or goal of history is the actualization of freedom in the life in the modern nation-state. He claimed that history was a rational process of development and that it could be understood and made intelligible for anyone willing to look at it rationally, which means looking at it holistically and as an endeavor of the world spirit with a discernible purpose.

Here I find a contradiction between human freedom and the world spirit or will. Is the world spirit G-d's or the holy human spirit? Only in the convergence or synthesis of the two is the contradiction resolved between the will of the Other and the freedom of the subject. But many in history have perished under this contradiction, either fighting against the Law or fighting against nature.

Moreover, Hegel attempted to show that history exhibited real progress toward the ultimate goal of freedom and that the modern period, the time in which he lived up until his death in 1831, brought this development to fruition and, in a way, a culmination. His awareness of history pointed to the end of history like the Bible does. This theory of history has been both highly influential and controversial – it is essential to any overall study of the philosophy of history.

The theory of history reflects Hegel's philosophy and dialectical method. The spirit dominates philosophy and history. A dominant king, or empire, is opposed by another nation with culture and ideals that are claimed to be dominant. Dominance and hegemony are not necessarily bad in that they may promote global development. The dominant country spends a large percentage of its budget on the military to maintain global peace. The United States is the world's police. Other nations then can spend money on development and catching up. This is the example of the United States and China. The United States spends money on the arms race, and China focuses on national defense.

China offers a good historical example where the peasants rebelled through armed struggle and oppressed the oppressors. Then to liberate the workers, the Communist Party established the dictatorship of the proletariat and went through purges of its own officials. Vietnam did the same and entered into a war of liberation with the United States.

Now do the people feel oppressed by a dictatorship? Not if it is a form of paternalism, and the growth, or wealth, of the people are emphasized. This is the case of China and Vietnam, but not of North Korea. China's gross domestic product grew at an amazing rate for 40 years thanks to free economic exchange and capitalism, not due to state-owned enterprises like the Soviet Union, which is no more.

So, the two systems combined rather than struggle and oppose one another. This is a good example of the dialectic of synthesis that is unopposed by an antithesis and ongoing struggle.

Now, previously, Hegel's student Karl Marx inverted Hegel's theory. For Hegel, the world spirit is what matters and how it influences a culture. The supra-structure determines the infrastructure, while for Marx it was the reverse: The infrastructure determines the supra-structure. You can be educated but live in dilapidated buildings and wear old clothes. In this China, emphasized how development is maximized through the building of great infrastructure, without too much ideological supra-structure. But without superstructure and freedom of ideas, they cannot innovate to higher levels of technology as in the West, despite having the talent. Talent requires innovation and freedom.

Hegel saw alienation and contradiction as necessary for development and progress. Culture alienates the animal or instinctual nature and socializes the young against their will. Marx instead interprets this as the dictatorships of the proletariat. The animal spirits must win and repress the divine spirits who exploited them and made them work. Marx did not understand a pure love for work and thought that this did not exist among the working class. But the mind state, or the superstructure, has a big influence on productivity and benevolent excess.

The late Marx saw impersonal bureaucratic structure and organization as necessary although alienating. In China, such communist bureaucracy worked in harmony with a traditional Chinese meritocracy and bureaucratic state organization. Finally, China did not struggle with America to develop, because America benefited from China's development.

Representative democracy unites the common sense of the many with the talent of the One, and this is a universally valid form of government. Talent, meritocracy, and rules by principles and ideas are the best form of government. The best people rule in the service of the people because they possess judgment, courage, justice, and moderation to the highest degree.

Socrates thought that the ambitions that drove most political leaders were a form of madness or a sickness of the soul. This perspective is entirely consistent with Darwin's and Freud's account of male leadership in the primal hoard. If justice is equality and rulers should be concerned with the welfare of their subjects rather than themselves, then justice promotes the interests of the weak not the strong, contrary to the animal spirits.

If we use this analysis to review what happened during the 2024 elections in the United States, we see that Trump's election victory is a victory of the less educated and blue-collar workers over the educated middle class and the educated rich. For years the Democratic Party privileged college education as a path from the working class to the middle and upper classes. However, the less educated felt diminished or left behind by this; plus, jobs were outsourced to other countries with lower wages and fewer worker protections.

Trump appears to favor the uneducated working classes but actually the working classes are supporting the tax cuts for the super-rich as if this benefitted them in some way. Trickle-down economics, or voodoo economics, as it is often called, claimed that lowering taxes for the rich would benefit the poor as well.

Trump is a man of no virtue and has been convicted of sexual abuse and assault and is a pathological liar. Even his riches are questionable. His lack of virtue was an advantage with his voters and led him to victory. He is very self-centered and thinks about himself before others. His followers love that vicariously and think of themselves as members of a superior great nation.

If G-d is the ruler of history, then a gentile with no virtue, has to be the anti-leader or the Antichrist. If G-d is not the ruler of history, then such is simply the product of karma, our impulses, and destructive passions. Such a figure does not exist in Judaism. Trump has no virtue, so he cannot be a savior despite what his followers think. In any case, according to Christianity, the true leader and the messianic world will come after the Antichrist.

How about that Trump is supporting the Christian value of pro-life and no abortions. Well, Christianity is the only religion that bases its faith on a prohibition on abortion. There's no prohibition on abortion in Judaism or Buddhism. This cannot be a universal value.

The major conflicts between capitalism and socialism have been resolved or reconciled, but how about the contemporary examples of Russia and Ukraine?

Russia invaded Ukraine with the imperial ambitions of the old czars and because some Russians living in Ukraine near the border with Russia want to be part of Russia. This implies that the fall of communism in the Soviet Union could lead to either liberalism (West Germany) or the emergence of Russian nationalism. The war is a war between autocratic Russian nationalism and a liberal political global order with established and recognized borders ratified by the United Nations.

What about colonialism, a term that has been so vilified in the West? Colonialism is the cultural aspect of an empire. This is something that the Mongol Empire, for example, did not have. Their empire was simply based on physical force and numbers. If an empire is not a civilization, then its grip on power will be short-lived.

First, an empire is built through military innovation. Then the empire imposes or brings its values to its colony. India became an English-speaking country and developed industry and the economy with the help of English values operating in harmony with traditional Indian values. This is why this form of empire is called a civilization.

A colony means a settlement leading to agriculture. The earth and animals are our colonized, but they both have developed and have been harmed by colonization.

Finally, there is the war between Arabs and Jews in Israel and its role in history. Both people are descendants of the Canaanites, but the Hebrews were made slaves in Egypt and later became Jews. God pointed to Israel as the promised land of the future Jews who were living in Canaan. They would go back to Canaan as Israel, not Canaan, but the other Canaanites and Palestinians remained there and either had to be killed or have their own country.

In this sense, this struggle in history is biblical. G-d promised Ishmael to make him a great nation but did not promise him a holy land like he did to Isaac's descendants. Both people are still fighting over the same land, but only one people have a right to inherit the land according to the Bible not to history if these two are not the same.

If G-d is the ruler of history and they are not intervening, this seems to confirm the theory that the dominant nation is the ruler of history. In the wars in the Bible, God is always determining which side will win based on their moral behavior. When Christians fight Muslims, and Muslims fight Jews because all three believe in the same monotheistic God, on which side of the war is God on? If you say the winning side, then there is no way of determining whether the war was won by God or humans. The victors are always the superior cause.

G-d and history seem to be helping Israel with its military technology. For the conflict to be resolved, both people need to accept a common border and a Jewish inheritance of the land. Muslims must renounce violence, while Christianity must abandon its claims to religious exclusivity (salvation only through Christ), which the new Catholic pope (Pope Francis) already has. Judaism must also embrace the brotherliness of humans and major religions.

Finally, the cyclical form of history has two views. First is repetition as trauma, genocide, and second, general suffering in history as destiny. The second is Tyche or destiny where humans struggle in repetitions that are therapeutic and lead to evolution, change, and enlightenment. This view of destiny does not conflict with the view of history and evolution as linear progress.

Now is history organized by various ideologies and discourses? What is the difference between ideology, science, religious texts, and discourse. For Lacanians, ideology is Imaginary and discourse is Symbolic. For example, in Genesis, G-d creates the material universe with symbolic words: 'Let there be Light'. The ideology is that G-d is a father in heaven that guides our development. The Symbolic discourse is that G-d does this with the law.

The rule of the king or master in history is the ideological form of the ruler of history or his earthly representative. If you are a Buddhist, for example, then the Buddhist is guided by ultimate reality or Buddha, but historically, Buddha did not get involved in government or political life. Buddha meditated and watched armies collide in war, but he did not try to stop them. How can a sacred wise consciousness, take sides in a violent struggle? From this point of view, how can G-d be the ruler of history?

The master (S_1) can be a spiritual master or a governmental or economic master (Plutarchy or the government of billionaires). S_2 is the ideology or teaching that is used to rule.

The Five Discourses

Lacan's theory of the five discourses for psychoanalysis was his attempt to formalize into mathematical ('mathemes') formulas the work of psychoanalysis and its relationship to culture and politics. Zizek has written a lot about this topic not being a practicing psychoanalyst himself.

In the practice of psychoanalysis, the practice is a talking cure for the analysand and a listening practice for the analyst. The patient is supposed to free-associate and speak freely without holding anything back. There's no discussion of politics, elections, or taking sides in their conflicts with their family. Psychoanalytic speech is more ‘chatting’ than intellectual discourse. This is why psychoanalysis is a science and politics is not.

Now what do ordinary people believe about discourse? I think people believe that language is important for social relationships and society, and they learn language in their relationships with their families and in school. So, what Lacan calls discourse refers to intellectual and scholarly discussions among teachers and students, scholars, and politicians. University discourse is not the same as the master’s or government’s discourse. Many ideas do not emerge in the university, but through experience, they challenge the beliefs taught in the university. Freud’s theory emerged from clinical professional practice. The university may choose to ignore him or develop his theory. The university discourse is really the discourse of natural science that rules the university.

In this sense, discourse is always related to power: who we speak to and what position we are as parent or student, teacher, and student, colonizer and colonized, capitalist and worker, or leader and subject. Here I present to you the five discourses.

Discourse of the Master	*Discourse of the University*
$\underline{S_1}\ \underline{S_2}$	$\underline{S_2} \rightarrow a$
$\$\ a$	$S_1 \rightarrow \$$
Discourse of the Hysteric	*Discourse of the Analyst*
$\underline{\$} \rightarrow S_1$	$a \rightarrow \underline{\$}$
$a\ S_2$	$S_2 \rightarrow S_1$
Discourse of the Capitalist	
$\underline{\$} \rightarrow \underline{S_2}$	
S_1 · A	

Terms

$: the divided subject or psychical *Spaltung*.

S_1= the master signifier of which there are two. First the signifier of the master or teacher, key terms, and words uttered. Second, when the signifier as the signified is in the body of jouissance it has a more profound impact.

S_2= the signified/signification in language and a dictionary. The Teaching

Objet a = the object cause of desire and there are six imaginary objects: breast, feces, phallus, hole, voice, gaze, and the ‘nothing’ or the agalma that is in the Real.

So far, I have been speaking of discourse as an intellectual capacity, but Lacan also speaks of discourse as a form of jouissance. Now jouissance is not a feeling but represents the pleasurable and painful aspect of feelings. Truth for Lacan always represents something enjoyable, but truth could also be painful to bear. The master is a transcendent ego that conforms to the myth of the ego ideal that dominates our actions. In this sense, the university discourse and the master's discourse always form a type of 'egocracy'. Here Lacan also speaks of G-d as jouissance more like the Buddha in Buddhism, rather than the Jewish God of the superego and the Mosaic law, although the rabbis also spoke of the joy of the law and they dance to it.

The formulas include four terms that are in various logical relations to each other of alternation, opposition, and subjugation. S_1 is the signifier, and S_2 is the signified or signification in language. S or $ is a divided subject. For Lacan's psycholinguistics, the subject is the same as and is defined by the signifier. The *objet a* is the object cause of desire. Lacan names several *objet a*: the breast, feces, the phallus or the hole, the voice, the gaze, and the agalma in the Real. *Objet a's* are imaginary and Real, while the signifier is symbolic.

As the discourse of the master or the government can be seen as ordinary social life, the discourse of the hysteric could also be called the discourse of psychopathology, or the discourse of suffering.

Finally, the discourse of the capitalist is the discourse where the subject completes himself or herself through consumption and scientific knowledge about the objects of consumption also leads to increased consumption. Lacan calls the *objet a* a 'lathouse' to refer to the use of computers and internet-based information and AI to impact consumption and economic exchange. The information about the *objet a* is Imaginary, but it facilitates economic exchange.

Appendix III

The Sinthome in Joyce, Lacan, and Jung

Contrary to Lacan (1975–1976b), who was interested and wrote about James Joyce's (1922) work, Jung actually met Joyce when he was treating his daughter for schizophrenia. When treating James Joyce's daughter, Lucia, Jung described her, and her father as "like two people going to the bottom of a river, one falling and the other diving": Jung believed that this comparison highlighted the distinction between the involuntary nature of psychosis ('falling') and the voluntary manifestation of the creative imagination ('diving').

I argue that Jung distinguished between the voluntary expression of the creative imagination and the involuntary nature of psychosis. Lacan instead argued that Joyce was saved or cured of psychosis by his literary writings, and by how he changed the structure of the English language to express his ideas. Jung only saw Lucia for a few sessions and put her under the care of Carey Baynes. He did not believe that Lucia could be cured. Joyce cured himself of his psychosis through writing. But was he a neurotic with perverse and psychotic features, or did he have a psychotic structure as Lacan believed.

Joyce was initially resistant to Jung's attempts to help Lucia gain distance from him. However, he later became more reconciled and respectful of Jung's assistance. Joyce inscribed Jung's copy of *Ulysses*.

In his autobiography *Memories, Dreams, and Reflections*, Jung (1961) reveals several aspects of himself and his work. He wrote this book at the end of his life. He was definitely an 'eidetic', 'mnemonist' person. His memory was large like the unconscious, and he read a large number of books constantly throughout his life. Jung's memory, more than his theory, is proof of his genius.

But this larger memory and eidetic thought came as an anxiety-producing or irrational imposition, as seen in delusions and obsessional ideation. However, as we know, the so-called normal neurotic also suffers from involuntary divisions and compulsions. Freud spoke of the *Spaltung* of consciousness.

Jung literally wrote in great detail about his personality 1 and 2 and his mother's personality 1 and 2. In addition, Jung (1961) for example spoke of the fear he had of the God that could not be named and always appeared alongside the friendly image of Jesus. Religion for Jung was something that he suffered or was done to him, contrary to the view of Jung as a religious man, like his father. Jung was not religious despite his interest in religion. His father, of course, was a Christian priest and scholar.

When he wrote he felt restless within an ominous atmosphere that was filled with ghostly entities. Then the writing began flowing out of him, and as soon as he took the pen, the room quieted and cleared. Jung's work shows how much modernity and modern science, as Jung called his work, still remained obfuscated by darker, more primitive forces.

In addition, Lacan says that in the case of psychosis, the supplementation and nomination provided by the sinthome (the fourth ring), coincides with the best results that can be expected from the practice of analysis. Since most analyses are of neurotics, who invariably retain some degree of character symptomatology after treatment, post analysis the symptom becomes a sintome or a teacher of the subject. For these reasons, I (Moncayo, 2017) have advanced the thesis that there are two knots of four (the first with untied rings and the second with the untied Imaginary), one for neurosis and one for psychosis.

In the knot of neurosis, the three rings are intrinsically tied together. Lacan says that in analysis the knot has to be untied. The knot needs to be re-knotted by the sinthome. In psychosis, the untied imaginary refers to the effect of the foreclosure of the name of the father. It is not that symptoms remain after treatment but that the illness needs to be cured by a new paternal metaphor, and that is what Lacan calls the sinthome. In the knot of four for psychosis the sinthome ties the imaginary to the other two while the imaginary still remains loose and untied.

In what I (Moncayo, 2017) call the sinthome or fourth ring for neurosis, the apparent psychotic symptoms (not structure) are a source of teaching for the subject.

This formulation should shed some light on the question raised by some whether Lacan, like Joyce, also had a psychotic structure for which his work was a sinthome. Most people seemed to agree that Jung suffered from episodes of psychosis, but otherwise, he had a conventional neurotic structure for his time. Lacan instead, like Joyce, was eccentric.

Jung, like Lacan (mostly), was self-analyzed while self-analysis in Lacanian analysis only begins after the personal analysis has ended. Self-analysis is not a personal analysis, because the analyst needs the Other to see their own unconscious. Neither Freud nor Jung was analyzed by an Other, and Lacan left his analysis with an ego psychologist before it was finished.

In addition, Jung suffered isolation in his self-analysis and at times could not work because of how disturbing his unconscious and his self-analysis were. He was flooded and almost broken by the unconscious. In his case, it was his unconscious, rather than other people, that proved to be disturbing. Jung's relationship with his father was neurotic because he admired him and loved him very much. Jung had a conventional neurotic structure with psychotic symptoms. Jung began his career as an expert in schizophrenia or dementia precox as it was called then. He gathered the material not from his practice as Freud did with hysteria but from his own analysis and method of working with his own unconscious.

Jung did not find the symptoms of psychosis strange or simply a biological malfunction, but phenomena that provided a lot of knowledge about the human mind. He thought that his writings were inspired by 'ghostly entities' around him. For a nonfunctional person, this would be considered a delusion.

Perhaps like in Joyce, according to Lacan, Jung's psychotic episodes helped a further exploration of the psyche that reorganized his modern Western psyche. But first his neurotic structure had to be undone through the return of repressed material that could lead to a new organization. In the end Jung died satisfied and happy with his life, contrary to Freud's cancer and pessimism at the time of his death.

In the case of Joyce, the sinthome exemplified by his writing was installed to prevent the precipitation of a psychotic disorder within what Lacan considered a psychotic structure. In the case of a psychotic disorder, the sinthome as a fourth element can be used to treat the symptoms of psychosis. The sinthome includes the illness, but the cure is not a part of the illness, although the illness also contributes to its own cure.

Bibiliography

APA Presidential Task Force. (2006, May–June). Evidence-Based Practice in Psychology. *American Psychologist.*

Augustine, S. (1958). *The City of God.* New York: Double Day Books.

Bateson, G. (1979). *Mind and Nature.* New York: Bentham Books.

Bion, W. (1963). *Elements of Psychoanalysis.* London: Heinemann Medical Books.

Bion, W. (1965). *Transformations.* London: Heinemann Medical Books.

Bion, W. (1970). *Attention and Interpretation.* London: Tavistock.

Bion, W. (1977). *A Memoir of the Future.* London: Karnac, 1990.

Bion, W. (1991). *Cogitations.* London: Karnac.

Borges, J. (2004). *The Aleph.* Emecé: Buenos Aires.

Cassirer, E. (1946). *Language and Myth.* New York: Dover Publications.

Eliade, M. (1949). *The Myth of the Eternal Return.* NJ: Princeton University Press.

Frege, G. (1892). *Meaning and Reference*, edited by A. W. Moore. New York: Oxford University Press, 1992.

Freud, S. (1933). New Introductory Lectures on Psychoanalysis. *SE*, 22, 3–182.

Harari, R. (1995). *How James Joyce Made His Name. A Reading of the Final Lacan.* The Other Press.

Hegel, G. H. (1822–1830). *Lectures on the Philosophy of World History.* London: Oxford University Press, 1975.

Hook, S. (1971). *Psychoanalysis, Scientific Method, and Philosophy.* New York: New York University Press, 2006.

Jones, E. (1916). *The Theory of Symbolism.* Presented before the Royal Society.

Joyce, J. (1922). *Ulysses.* New York: Dover Publications.

Jung, C. G. (1961). *Memories, Dreams, Reflections.* New York: Vintage Books.

Jung, C. G. (2009). *The Red Book.* New York: Norton, and Norton.

Kristeva, J. (1941). *Desire in Language.* New York: Columbia University Press, 1980.

Lacan, J. (1969–1970). *The Underside of Psychoanalysis.* New York: Norton & Norton, 2007.

Lacan, J. (1964). *The Four Fundamental Concepts of Psychoanalysis.* New York: Norton, and Norton, 1981.

Lacan, J. (1975–1976a). *The Seminar of Jacques Lacan, Book XXIII*, edited by J.-A. Miller. Cambridge: Polity Press, 2016.

Lacan, J. (1975–1976b). *The Sinthome. The Seminar of Jacques Lacan, Book XXIII*. London: Polity Press.
Lacan, J. (2016). . . . *o peor. Seminario XIX*. Buenos Aires: Paidos.
Langs, R. (1998a). *Current Theories of Psychoanalysis*. Madison, CT: International University Press.
Langs, R. (1998b). *Ground Rules in Psychotherapy and Counselling*. London: Karnac Books.
Langs, R., Baladamenti, A. and Thomson, L. (1996). *The Cosmic Cycle: The Unification of Mind, Matter, and Energy*. Brooklyn, NY: Alliance.
Leibniz, G. W. (1898). *The Theodicy*. Leipzig: Open Court, 1902.
Leichsenring, F. and Rabung, S. (2008). Effectiveness of Long-Term Psychodynamic Psychotherapy: A Meta-Analysis. *Journal of the American Medical Association*, 300, 1551–1565.
Leichsenring, F. and Rabung, S. (2009). Analyzing Effectiveness of Long-Term Psychodynamic Psychotherapy Reply. *The Journal of the American Medical Association*, 301, 932–933.
Levy, R. A., Ablon, J. S. and Kächele, H. (2011). *Psychodynamic Psychotherapy Research: Evidence-Based Practice and Practice-Based Evidence*. Springer, Kindle Edition.
Locke, J. (1632–1704). *An Essay Concerning Human Understanding*. Cambridge: Hackett Publishing Company.
Matte-Blanco, I. (1975). *The Unconscious as Infinite Sets. An Essay in Bi-Logic*. London: Karnac.
Miller, J. A. (2015). *Pure Psychoanalysis, Applied Psychoanalysis, and Psychotherapy*. www.lacan.com/lacinkXX2.htm. Accessed February 2015.
Moncayo, R. (2017). *Lalangue, Sinthome, Jouissance, and Nomination. A Reading Companion and Commentary on Lacan's Seminar XXIII on the Sinthome*. London: Karnac.
Moncayo, R. and Romanowicz, M. (2015). The Real Jouissance of Uncountable Numbers. London: Karnac.
Moncayo, R. (2018). *Knowing, Not-Knowing, and Jouissance*. London: Palgrave.
Muller, J. P. (1996). *Beyond the Psychoanalytic Dyad. Developmental Semiotics in Freud, Pierce, and Lacan*. New York: Routledge.
Nobus, D. and Quinn, M. (2005). *Knowing Nothing, Staying Stupid*. London: Routledge.
Plotnitsky, A. (2000). *On Lacan and Mathematics*. New York: Other Press.
Plotnitsky, A. (2002). *The Knowable and the Unknowable*. Ann Arbor: University of Michigan Press.
Plotnitsky, A. (2009). On Lacan and Mathematics. *Oeuvres & Critiques*, XXXIV. https://torontopsychoanalysis.com/about-us/ispsychoanalysis effective/#:~:text=A%20review%20of%2014%20good,disorders%20and%20general%20psychosocial%20functioning. Accessed 18 January 2023.
Robson, A. L. (2002). Critical/Sensitive Periods. In Salkind, N. J. (ed.). *Child Development. Gale Virtual Reference Library*. New York: Macmillan Reference USA, pp. 101–103.
Scholem, G. (1991). *On the Mystical Head of the Godhead*. New York: Schocken Books.
Zizek, S. (2000). *The Fragility of the Absolute*. London: Verso.

Index

Note: Page numbers in *italic* indicate a figure and page numbers in **bold** indicate a table on the corresponding page.

For Product Safety Concerns and Information please contact our EU representative GPSR@taylorandfrancis.com Taylor & Francis Verlag GmbH, Kaufingerstraße 24, 80331 München, Germany

Printed and bound by CPI Group (UK) Ltd, Croydon, CR0 4YY
14/09/2026
02216223-0009